Living Skills Recovery Workbook

Living Skills Recovery Workbook

Pat Precin, MS, OTR
Director of Occupational, Recreational, and Creative Arts Therapies, St. Luke's-Roosevelt Hospital, New York; *Consultant*, Private Practice, New York

Foreword by

Tina Barth, MA, OTR/L, CRC
Adjunct Faculty, Department of Occupational Therapy, Touro College and City University of New York, New York

Butterworth Heinemann

Boston Oxford Auckland Johannesburg Melbourne New Delhi

A member of the Reed Elsevier group

Every effort has been made to ensure that the drug dosage schedules within this text are accurate and conform to standards accepted at time of publication. However, as treatment recommendations vary in the light of continuing research and clinical experience, the reader is advised to verify drug dosage schedules herein with information found on product information sheets. This is especially true in cases of new or infrequently used drugs.

Recognizing the importance of preserving what has been written, Butterworth–Heinemann prints its books on acid-free paper whenever possible.

AMERICAN FORESTS GLOBAL RELEAF 2000

Butterworth–Heinemann supports the efforts of American Forests and the Global ReLeaf Program in its campaign for the betterment of trees, forests, and our environment.

Library of Congress Cataloging-in-Publication Data
ISBN 0-7506-7118-1

British Library Cataloguing-in-Publication Data
A catalogue record for this book is available from the British Library.

The publisher offers special discounts on bulk orders of this book.
For information, please contact:

Manager of Special Sales
Butterworth–Heinemann
225 Wildwood Avenue
Woburn, MA 01801-2041
Tel: 781-904-2500
Fax: 781-904-2620

For information on all B–H medical publications available, contact our World Wide Web home page at: http://www.bh.com

10 9 8 7 6 5 4 3 2

Printed in the United States of America

Dedicated to all the people who have shared their lives and opened their hearts in order to better themselves.

Contents

Foreword

Mentally ill chemically addicted (MICA) persons are fully addicted and fully mentally ill at the same time. In MICA situations there are two diseases occurring together and they have an effect on each other. The author confronts the difficulty of addressing both diseases concurrently through a program to improve coping skill capacity. The exercises are written simply, taking the concrete thinking often present in mental illness and early sobriety into account. Coping skill development is presented as increasing the probability of success in recovery. The workbook program targets improvement in coping skills in time management, stress management, social skills, and activities of daily living.

The author addresses difficult questions through the design of her program and its feedback loops. How is it possible to face a problem while being helpless and feeling overwhelmed? How is it possible to promote flexible problem solving in a highly defended, rigid, concrete-thinking person? What is the relationship of the person receiving services to the person delivering the services? Where does self-help fit into this model?

There is a requirement for personal responsibility and action built into the 12 steps that underlie the self-help movement. The clinical challenge is to help recovering persons to make the intellectual and emotional commitment to recovery and to develop the skills to take the necessary actions on their own.

This workbook gives detailed lesson plans for helping recovering people to develop or strengthen the underlying skills needed to cope with life while getting sober and maintaining sobriety. In true 12-step fashion the workbook recognizes that recovery comes from individual work and shared experience. It is designed to be used by recovering people alone, with others or with a clinical staff. The quality assurance studies help the recovering person assess his current skill level and plan the next step in skill building. These studies can also be used to demonstrate the recovering person's progress in achieving outcomes as a measure of the clinical effectiveness of a treatment program.

It is wonderful to see this practical occupational therapy approach so clearly presented and made available to other professions and directly to the consumers themselves.

Tina Barth

Preface

HOW THIS BOOK CAME ABOUT

My first exposure to life skills in psychoeducation training with psychiatric clients (consumers) came from the therapeutic activities department of Payne Whitney clinic where I was employed as an occupational therapist. Here, Susan Fine, M.A., OTR, FAOTA, and Perri Schwimmer-Stern, Ed.D., Ph.D., had written a life skills treatment manual which was implemented in the clinic for years to come. The value of skills training to psychiatric consumers[1] was foremost in my mind as I later began work in a dual diagnosis outpatient program for substance abusing psychiatric consumers at St. Luke's-Roosevelt Hospital. (This same setting is often referred to as a MICA program standing for "Mentally Ill and Chemically Addicted.") The patient population was composed of substance abusers who also had a major psychotic disorder on Axis I. Most were chronically and persistently mentally ill. Most had a history of forensic involvement, homelessness, medical problems associated with long-term substance abuse, and poor or no social supports. Many had already been through the system—detoxifications, rehabilitation, day treatment programs for psychiatric illnesses—but continued to relapse and/or become symptomatic. Two thirds of the population had cognitive deficits.[2,3] With few exceptions, most could not work.

The dual diagnosis program had originally begun as a clinic where patients were seen one time per week by a social worker for psychotherapy and for work in their recovery, and by a psychiatrist to receive medication as needed. Over a six-year period the program incorporated treatment groups run by occupational therapists, creative arts therapists, psychologists, nurses, and substance abuse counselors, becoming a state of the art program in New York City.

At this time, I arrived on board and noticed several trends in treatment at St. Luke's and in other dual diagnosis programs. First, living skills were taught separately from substance abuse issues and were absent in double trouble groups which usually address medication, the effects of substance abuse on mental health problems and vice versa, and the symptoms of both illnesses. Second, "conventional 12-step groups alone lacked acquisitional skills training necessary for developing effective coping mechanisms."[4] Third, psychoeducational living skills groups were heavily based in social skills training even though MICA consumers may present with profound deficits in volitional and adaptive components as well.[5–9]

If living skills are taught without an emphasis on recovery, consumers may develop functional skills over an underlying addiction process. "If such living skills are built over the addiction disease, the new skills will become weak and ineffective as the addiction process takes over."[4]

Furthermore, MICA consumers have been shown to demonstrate concrete versus abstract thinking, and deficits in memory, judgment, and attention.[2,3] These cognitive problems may make it difficult for them to learn and recall new information, and generalize it to other treatment groups or to their outside lives. So, it is not enough to have a dual diagnosis program with groups for skills training separate from groups for substance abuse. Both the skill training and recovery need to be tightly coupled and taught simultaneously.

Keeping in mind current treatment trends, cognitive impairments, characteristic problems of the population, and current changes in the mental health care system (managed care), I wrote the *Living Skills Recovery Workbook*. It incorporates stress management, time management, activities of daily living, and social skills training with 12-step practices. "Each living skill is taught with relationship to how it aids in recovery and relapse prevention for each consumer's individual lifestyle, living situation, and pattern of addiction. This form of treatment may allow MICA consumers to learn and use the necessary skills to become and remain drug free and to manage their psychiatric symptoms to promote the highest level of integration into their community."[10]

The skills training modules were based on the Liberman[11] approach but needed to be modified. Less written material was used, as our consumers have an average reading level of sixth grade. Instead, more personal accounts of the material being learned were used. Material was graded more, to meet the needs of the individuals yet still be conducive to group settings.

Daley has published a workbook[12] and training guide[13] for dual diagnosis consumers. His material is highly textual and may be appropriate for substance abusers with a mental illness who are more psychiatrically stable, have a high capacity for insight into their illnesses, read and write on an advanced level, and are higher functioning. The *Living Skills Recovery Workbook* can be used to treat consumers who are either illiterate or literate. It is geared towards people who are chronically ill and may have less insight into their illnesses.

The *Living Skills Recovery Workbook* is unique in that it contains its own easy-to-use quality assurance study. Consumers can use it to check their progress on a daily basis. Clinicians can use it for treatment justification and publications. The objectives for each exercise can be used as treatment goals, making documentation less time-consuming. The workbook's effectiveness has been statistically studied over a three-year period at the St. Luke's-Roosevelt Hospital with successful outcomes.

WHO THIS BOOK IS FOR

This book can be used by providers, consumers, educators, students, and managed care companies, all of whom are involved with the treatment and management of consumers who suffer from both an addiction and a mental illness. Most of the exercises are geared towards MICA consumers; however, some exercises are also appropriate for substance abusers only, and some for consumers afflicted solely with mental illness.

Prevalence of Concurrent Chemical Abuse and Mental Illness

The comorbidity of chemical abuse–dependency and psychiatric disorders as defined on Axis I of *DSM IV*[14] is very high, although the percentages may vary according to nosologic criteria, social trends, assessment techniques, and location.[15–18] Of the general population 17% are diagnosed as MICA.[15,16] One study found that 87% of people diagnosed with a primary mental disorder also had a secondary diagnosis of alcohol abuse or dependence.[19] Of the total psychiatric population in treatment, up to 50% will also have a diagnosis of substance abuse–dependence.[15,20,21,22] More specifically the percentages of people who have secondary diagnoses of substance abuse–dependence are:

- 84% of people with antisocial and borderline personality disorders.[15,20]
- 47–65% of people with schizophrenia (lifetime estimate).[15,16]
- 50% of people with schizoaffective disorders.[15,20]
- 30% of people with major depression.[15,20]
- 28% of people with anxiety disorders.[15,20]
- 25% of people with bipolar illness.[15,20]

SETTINGS THIS BOOK CAN BE USED IN

This book can be used in:

- outpatient MICA programs
- intensive outpatient services
- intensive psychiatric rehabilitation treatment programs (IPRTs)
- MICA groups
- shelters
- consumer groups
- home care assertive community treatment (ACT) teams
- private clinics
- inpatient detoxification units
- libraries
- drug and alcohol certification programs
- 12-step groups
- private practices
- adolescent after school programs
- prevention programs
- settings that treat battered women and sexual abuse
- obsessive-compulsive disorder clinics
- HMOs
- outpatient psychiatric day treatment programs
- partial hospitalization programs
- continuing day treatment programs (CDTPs)
- double trouble groups
- supported residences
- peer support groups
- ambulatory detoxification units
- inpatient psychiatric units
- homes of clients
- in schools that teach about substance abuse and mental illness
- business employee assistance programs (EAPs)
- state hospitals
- family therapy centers
- high schools
- settings that deal with the treatment of autoimmunological deficiency syndrome (AIDS)
- settings that treat other types of addictions
- anxiety clinics
- a variety of managed care settings

OBJECTIVES FOR WRITING THIS BOOK

This book was written to:

1. Improve quality of life and productivity in society by helping people manage their addictions and psychiatric symptoms.
2. Provide a treatment that is flexible enough to be used in a variety of settings, for different lengths of treatment and by different disciplines, yet addresses core issues of MICA clients.
3. Provide a method for independent study so consumers can help themselves, in addition to other forms of treatment as necessary.

4. Provide a training tool to universities and certification programs. The workbook can be used as a textbook in the classroom, and then used in the clinic during an internship. This may help integrate theoretical knowledge and clinical practice. It may also decrease the anxiety of the students in the clinical setting because the book is already familiar to them.
5. Provide an easy-to-use quality assurance measure for MICA treatment.
6. Provide preventative treatment to decrease costly inpatient stays.
7. Provide a workbook for consumer run self-help groups.

WHY THIS BOOK IS NEEDED

This book is needed to teach consumers concretely how each living skill is necessary to one's own personal recovery from addiction. For example, when discussing how to structure free time, a common approach may be to do an activity interest check list, followed by an activity analysis, followed by setting a goal to incorporate the new activity into one's schedule. In this new approach the following additional points would be emphasized:

1. How the particular activity chosen may help the consumer regain some control over his or her life that addiction has taken away.
2. The activity chosen would be one directly related to their pattern of addiction.
   a. It should be available in or nearby their dwelling to be used when cravings arise. This way, they will engage in a purposeful activity instead of using drugs or alcohol.
   b. It would help manage their personal triggers that usually cause them to use drugs or alcohol. For example, if the trigger is loneliness, then the activity would be a social one involving people who are not involved in the addiction. If the trigger is having too much time on their hands, the activity would be long in duration. If the trigger is being overwhelmed with too much responsibility, the activity would be simple, pleasurable, and relaxing.
3. A discussion may take place around the need for immediate gratification, how this relates to the activity and how it relates to addiction.
4. A discussion around how working on recovery is not just constantly dealing with problems, but it is also learning to get pleasure out of nondrug-related activities, which build self-esteem and allow the consumer to begin to forgive themselves for wrongs they feel they have done during their drug use.

5. A discussion around how drugs and alcohol can take over all of one's time and energy, and how the same energy that was once used in the pursuit of drugs and alcohol can now be used productively if structured.

It is believed that the combination of living skills and recovery in the same session will increase both the likelihood of follow-through with goals and the likelihood of becoming or remaining drug free.

Pat Precin

REFERENCES

1. Fine, S. B., and Schwimmer, P. The effects of occupational therapy on independent living skills. The American Occupational Therapy Association, *Mental Health Special Interest Section Newsletter*, 9(4) (Dec. 1986).
2. Harrison, T. S., and Precin, P. Cognitive impairments in clients with dual diagnosis (chronic psychotic disorders and substance abuse): considerations for treatment. *Occupational Therapy International*, 3(2) (1996): 122–141.
3. Meek, P., Clark, H., and Solana, V. Neurocognitive impairment: the unrecognized component of dual diagnosis in substance abuse treatment. *J of Psychoactive Drugs*, 21 (1989): 153–160.
4. Precin, P. Living skills for recovery: A new occupational therapy approach for mentally ill chemical abusers (MICA). In *Sharing a global perspective: Book of abstracts.* Montreal: Twelfth International Congress of the World Federation of Occupational Therapists, 1998, C54.(Abstr.).
5. Corrigan, P. W., Schade, M. L., and Liberman, R. P. Social skills training. In Liberman, R.P. (ed.), *Handbook of psychiatric rehabilitation.* Boston: Allyn and Bacon, 1992, pp. 95–126.
6. Evans, K., and Sullivan, J. M. *Dual Diagnosis: Counseling the Mentally Ill Substance Abuser.* New York: Guilford Press, 1990, pp. 1–11.
7. Pensker, H. Addicted patients in hospital psychiatric units. *Psychiatric Annals* 13 (1983): 619–623.
8. Trier, T. R., and Levy, R. J. Emergency, urgent and elective admissions: Studies in a general hospital psychiatric emergency service. *Archives of General Psychiatry* 21 (1969): 423–430.
9. Perkins, K. A., Simpson, J. C., and Tsuang, M. T. Ten year follow-up of drug abusers with acute or chronic psychosis. *Hospital and Community Psychiatry* 37(5) (1986): 481–484.
10. Precin, P. Living skills for recovery: A new approach for mentally ill chemical abusers (MICA). In *Proceedings for the Twelfth*

International Congress of the World Federation of Occupational Therapists. Montreal: WFOT, in press.

11. Liberman, R. P. *Social and Independent Living Skills. Basic Conversation Skills Module. Workbook.* Los Angeles, CA: Clinical Research Center for Schizophrenia and Psychiatric Rehabilitation, UCLA, 1990, pp. 1–119.
12. Daley, D. C. *Dual Diagnosis Workbook. Recovery Strategies for Addiction and Mental Health Problems.* Independence, MO: Herald House/Independence Press, 1994, pp. 1–163.
13. Daley, D. C., and Thase, M. E. *Dual Disorders Recovery Counseling: A Biopsychosocial Treatment Model for Addiction and Psychiatric Illness.* Independence, MO: Herald House/Independence Press, 1994, pp. 1–170.
14. American Psychiatric Association. *Diagnostic and Statistical Manual of Mental Disorders*, 4th ed. Washington, D.C.: American Psychiatric Press, 1994.
15. Regier, D. A., Farmer, M. E., Rae, D. S., et al. Comorbidity of mental disorders with alcohol and other drug abuse. *JAMA* 264 (19) (1990): 2511–2518.
16. Mueser, K. T., Bellack, A. S., and Blanchard, J. J. Comorbidity of schizophrenia and substance abuse: implications for treatment. *J of Consulting and Clinical Psychology* 60 (6) (1992): 845–856.
17. Test, M. A., Knoedler, W. H., Allness, D. J., et al. Characteristics of young adults with schizophrenic disorders treated in the community. *Hospital and Community Psychiatry* 36 (1985): 853–858.
18. Test, M. A., Wallisch, L., Allness, D. J., et al. Substance use in young adults with schizophrenic disorders. *Schizophrenia Bulletin* 15 (1989): 465–476.
19. Kiesler, C. A., Simpkins, C. G., and Morton, T. L. Prevalence of dual diagnosis of mental and substance abuse disorders in general hospitals. *Hosp Community Psychiatry* 42 (4) (1991): 400–403.
20. Helzer, J. E., and Przybeck, T. R. The co-occurence of alcoholism with other psychiatric disorders in general population and its impact on treatment. *J Stud Alcohol* 49 (1988): 219–224.
21. Miller, N. S. *Comorbidity of psychiatric and alcohol/drug disorders: interactions and independent status. J of Addictive Diseases*, 12 (3) (1993): 5–16. Also published in *Comorbidity of Addictive and Psychiatric Disorders*, ed. by Miller, N. S., and Stimmel, B., Binghampton, NY: Haworth Press, 1993, pp. 5–16.
22. Kosten, T. R., and Kleber, H. D. Differential diagnosis of psychiatric comorbidity in substance abusers. *J Sub Abuse Treat* 5 (1988): 201–206.

Acknowledgments

I would like to thank the following people and organizations for their support in creating this book. I am grateful to the staff and clients of the dual diagnosis program, the inpatient detoxification units, and Clark 8 of St. Luke's-Roosevelt Hospital, New York, for continuously helping me gain insight into the nature of dual diagnosis. I would like to thank Dr. Hugh Cummings for his belief in and promotion of this type of treatment. My sincere appreciation goes to my boss, Cheryl King, for encouraging the publication of this work. Many thanks to my occupational therapy students: Margie Gaydos, Aimee Targovnick, Deepa Solomon, Rosalee Howell, Richard Sabel, Colleen Petak, Lisa Wiesen, Maria Kupershteyn, Terri Harrison, Kris Hagen, and others who used the material in their treatment groups, collected quality assurance data, helped refine the material, and moved the book towards publication. Research studying the efficacy of the *Living Skills Recovery Workbook* in the treatment of dual diagnoses clients was supported by a grant from the Metropolitan New York District of the New York State Occupational Therapy Association. I would also like to thank Sigurd Ackerman for promoting further research. Statistical guidance was provided by Ilene Wilets, Quihu Shi, and Arthur Blank of Beth Israel Hospital, New York; and Margaret Ferick of St. Luke's-Roosevelt Hospital, New York. I am grateful to Celeste Nieves for word processing and Peter LaBarbera for emotional support. The graphic designs were reproduced from Power Point 4.0. And finally, I thank Karen Oberheim, Jana Friedman, Leslie Kramer, and Mary Drabot of Butterworth–Heinemann for their patience and production of this book.

All material adapted from Perri Schwimmer-Stern, Ed.D., Ph.D., was part of a project developed with Susan Fine, M.A., OTR, FAOTA, at the Payne Whitney Clinic-New York Hospital.

1 Introduction

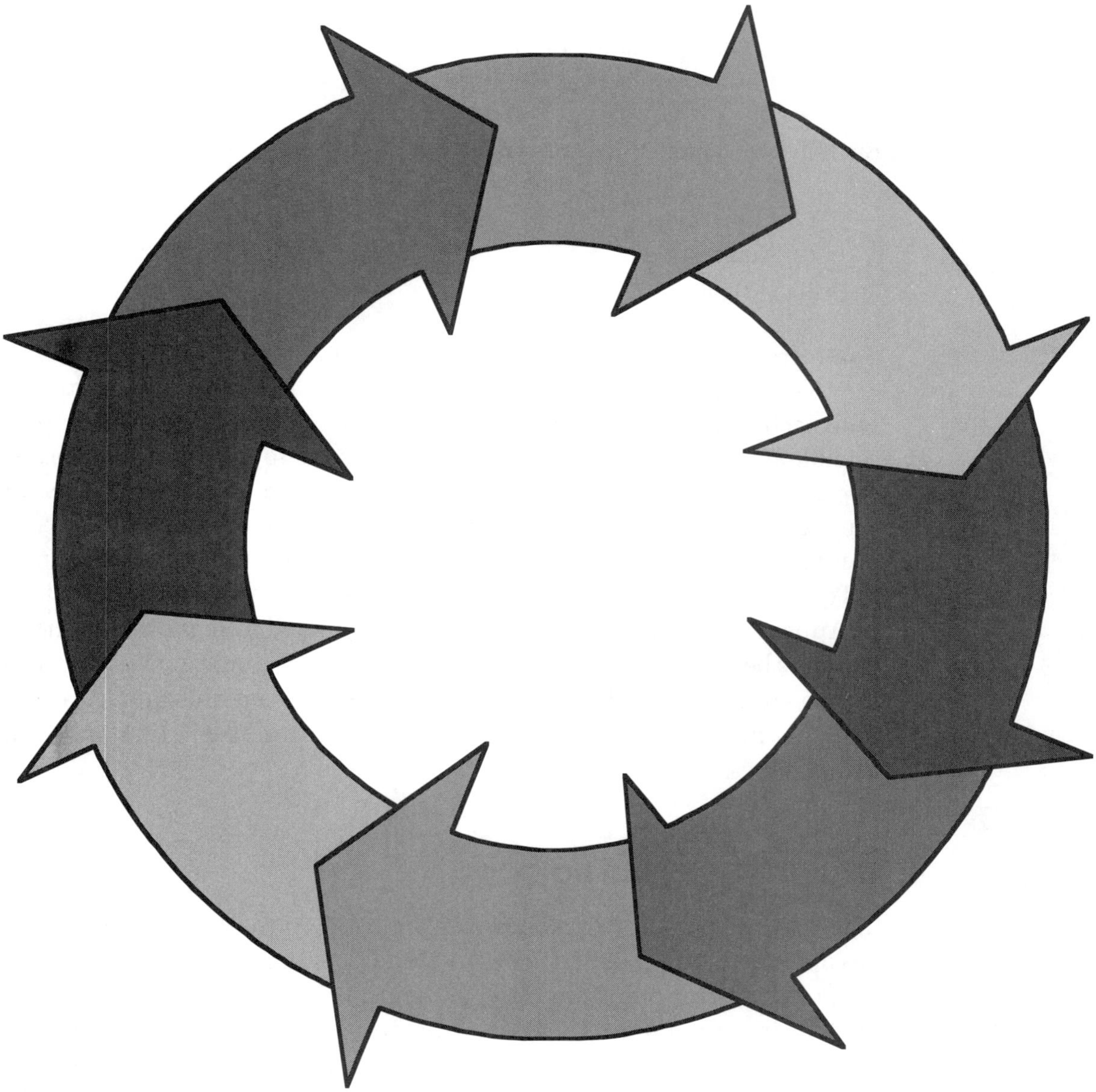

LAYOUT OF THE WORKBOOK

This book is divided into four *topic areas* (chapters):

1. Time Management for 12-Step Treatment.
2. Stress Management for Recovery.
3. Social Skills for Sobriety.
4. Activities of Daily Living for Abstinence.

Each topic area is divided into approximately sixteen different *sessions* related to the particular topic area. Each session is divided into two parts:

1. A Group Leader Plan.
2. Forms.

Each group leader plan contains three sections:

1. Objectives.
2. Materials.
3. Procedures.

Some group leader plans contain homework.

The purpose of the group leader plan is to explain how to proceed with each session, including how to complete the forms. Forms are reproducible handouts. A session may contain one, two, three, or four forms, depending on the session. A few sessions do not contain any forms. In these cases, the material for discussion is presented verbally, on a board, or involves different techniques such as role playing or therapeutic games. All of these are described in each group leader plan. There are also sessions in Appendix 1. These sessions have been separated from the others in the chapters because they are common to all four of the topic areas. They also have a group leader plan and forms. Appendix 2 contains quality assurance material. There is also a glossary of 12-step terms that are used throughout this book.

HOW TO USE THIS BOOK

The material in the workbook can be used in total or in part. Each session was written so it can stand alone. It is therefore possible to use just one session one time only, for a group of consumers in settings such as inpatient detoxification units, inpatient psychiatric units, partial hospitalizations, or community psychiatric emergency programs where the length of stay is short. If more time is available for treatment, multiple sessions can be given or complete topic areas (chapters) covered in settings such as consumer peer support groups, outpatient programs, 12-step groups, or residential environments. It is also possible to begin a consumer on one session in treatment and have him or her complete the rest of the material on their own, showing you their results. This may work in clinic settings where case management is provided. It is not necessary to follow the order of the workbook; however, a logical order is provided if one so chooses. A logical order would be as follows:

1. Introduction (Appendix 1).
2. Pre-quiz (Appendix 2).
3. Defining the Topic Area (Appendix 1).
4. Individual Sessions as Ordered in the Workbook (Chapters 2–5).
5. Review of the Topic Areas (Appendix 1).
6. Post-quiz (Appendix 2).
7. Topic Evaluation (Appendix 2).
8. QA Data Sheet (optional) (Appendix 2).
9. Graduation (Appendix 1).

The above order would be repeated for each of the four topic areas if the workbook was to be used in its entirety.

This book can be used in a group setting, in a one-to-one setting, or by a consumer independently.

For Self-Help Study by an Individual Consumer

Read the Preface and the Introduction to get an idea of what the book is about. Look in the table of contents and circle the sessions that you want help with. If you are not sure what sessions you may need help with, take each pretest and score yourself for each topic area. If you find that you did not answer most of them correctly, you may wish to study that topic area. Prioritize the sessions according to your needs. You may skip around or go in order, but finish each session before moving on to another one.

For each session read the group leader plan before you begin filling out the "forms" for that session. The "objectives" are guidelines which let you know what to accomplish in each session. The "materials" tell you what you will need, in most cases they are a pen and the workbook. Disregard any statements about the group, since you are working individually. Follow the "procedures." Try to be as honest as possible, because this work is for you. If you complete an entire topic area, you may wish to retake the quiz and compare your score with your previous score before you begin the next topic. The most important outcome is to be able to use this information to make positive changes in your life.

One-to-One Treatment

Use the table of contents to identify which sessions are of importance to the treatment. Prioritize the sessions and develop a treatment goal for completing them. The session leader should read the group leader plan before the treatment session begins to get an idea of how to guide the consumer through that session. During the session, follow the "procedures," ignoring statements about group members since only the two of you are working together. Give feedback to the consumer about how they did on each session.

Group Setting

The table of contents may be copied and handed out. The group members could then circle the number of each session they would like to work on in the group. The group leader decides with the help of the group which sessions will be addressed and which topic areas will be covered. Sessions can progress in order or by skipping around. It is recommended that each topic area be defined first (see session on definitions in Appendix 1).

In determining how to best use this book in your setting, a needs assessment on the population to be treated may be helpful. It may include the following information:

1. How many consumers at your setting currently need this treatment?
2. How much time does each consumer have for this treatment?
3. Which consumers wish to work on/need Time Management for 12-Step Treatment, Social Skills for Sobriety, ADL for Abstinence, Stress Management for Recovery, or a combination of the above?

HOW TO USE THE APPENDICES

Appendix 1 contains sessions which are pertinent to all of the four topic areas.

Introduction: This session introduces the workbook and states how it may be helpful.

Defining "Time Management," "Stress Management," "Social Skills," and "Activities for Daily Living": This session helps consumers define each topic area and demonstrate their current knowledge and skill level of each.

Goal Setting: The goal setting sheet may be copied and used throughout all of the sessions whenever a consumer wishes to set a goal. Setting goals frequently is desirable because it helps reinforce the newly learned material and helps generalize the skills to the person's life outside the treatment rooms. It also gives the person and/or provider feedback within a week (short-term goal) to help him or her gauge if the material was comprehended. The goal should be related to the session that was just completed. For best results, only one goal should be set at a time. It is helpful to use the same sheet for goal setting over and over again to reinforce the underlying equation of goal setting no matter what the content of the goal. Over time, this equation may become ingrained in the person's way of thinking so that they can set goals in their heads and the sheet becomes less necessary.

Review: The review session reinforces information and skills from previous session. Repetition of material has been thought to enhance skill acquisition and learning.[1–3]

Graduation: The graduation session provides a forum for additional feedback and celebration of accomplishment.

Appendix 2 contains quality assurance material.

Quizzes: There are four quizzes, one for each topic area. There are four group leader plans which contain the answers to each quiz. To measure progress, one quiz can be given before starting the topic area (prequiz) then readministered after completion of that topic area (postquiz). The difference in scores measures the ability to learn, store, and recall psychoeducational material.

Topic Evaluations: This session requests consumer feedback about each topic area. It provides information on whether or not the consumer(s) report having learned new material and/or made changes in their lives as a result of this treatment.

Quality Assurance Data Sheet: This session provides a summary sheet for collecting efficacy data and a group leader plan explaining how to use it. If a QA study is to be done, it will be helpful to read this session before beginning treatment, as data is easier to collect from the beginning.

LANGUAGE

Twelve-step language is used throughout this book whenever possible. There are many reasons for this:

1. Many MICA clients have difficulty attending 12-step groups on the outside. One of the ways to make it easier for consumers to feel comfortable in 12-step groups is to use the same language that is familiar to them from their MICA program, or vice versa.
2. Using a common language helps reinforce common issues of recovery between treatment groups, between treatment settings, and between providers and consumers. The familiarity and consistency brings trust and may decrease anxiety.
3. Repetition of certain words and key phrases has been thought to increase attention span and memory for the material.[4,5]

There is a glossary of 12-step terms used in this workbook towards the end of the book. It is recommended that providers become comfortable speaking this language to consumers, and help consumers understand the meaning of each concept as it relates to their own recovery.

RESULTS OF A THREE-YEAR STUDY

The effectiveness of the *Living Skills Recovery Workbook* was examined over a three-year period in the dual diagnosis program of St. Luke's-Roosevelt Hospital in New York City. The patient population was the same as described earlier. The sample size was 99. The effectiveness was measured against a control group who were also treated in the same dual diagnosis program, but did not receive the *Living Skills Recovery Workbook* treatment.

Results showed that MICA consumers made significant improvements in their living skills.[6] MICA consumers that received *Living Skills Recovery Workbook* treatment had significantly more clean time or fewer relapses than their control group.[6] MICA consumers significantly increased their clean time during and after receiving the treatment as compared to their previous amount of clean time before treatment in three out of the four topic areas.[6]

All results above were significant at the $p < .05$ level. The study was funded in part by the Metropolitan New York District of the New York State Occupational Therapy Association. Complete results of the study will be submitted for journal publication.

REFERENCES

1. Liberman, R. P., Mueser, K. T., Wallace, C. J., Jacobs, H. E., Echman, T., and Massel, H. K. Training skills in the psychiatrically disabled: Learning coping and competence. *Schizophrenia Bulletin* 12 (1986): 631–647.
2. Mueser, K. T., Bellack, A. S., Douglas, M. S., and Wade, J. H. Prediction of social skill acquisition in schizophrenic and major affective disorder patients from memory and symptomatology. *Psychiatry Research* 37 (1991): 281–296.
3. Oltmanns, T. F. Selective attention in schizophrenic and manic psychoses: The effect of distraction on information processing. *Journal of Abnormal Psychology* 87 (1987): 212–225.
4. Corrigan, P. W., Schade, M. L., and Liberman, R. P. Social skills training. In Liberman, R. P. (ed.), *Handbook of Psychiatric Rehabilitation.* Boston: Allyn and Bacon, 1992, pp. 95–126.
5. Toglia, J. Attention and memory. In Royeen, C. (ed.), *AOTA Self Study Series: Cognitive Rehabilitation.* Rockville, MD: AOTA, 1993, pp. 1–18.
6. Precin, P. Living skills for recovery: A new approach for Mentally Ill Chemical Abusers (MICA). In *Proceedings for the Twelfth International Congress of the World Federation of Occupational Therapists.* Montreal: WFOT, in press.

2 Time Management for 12-Step Treatment

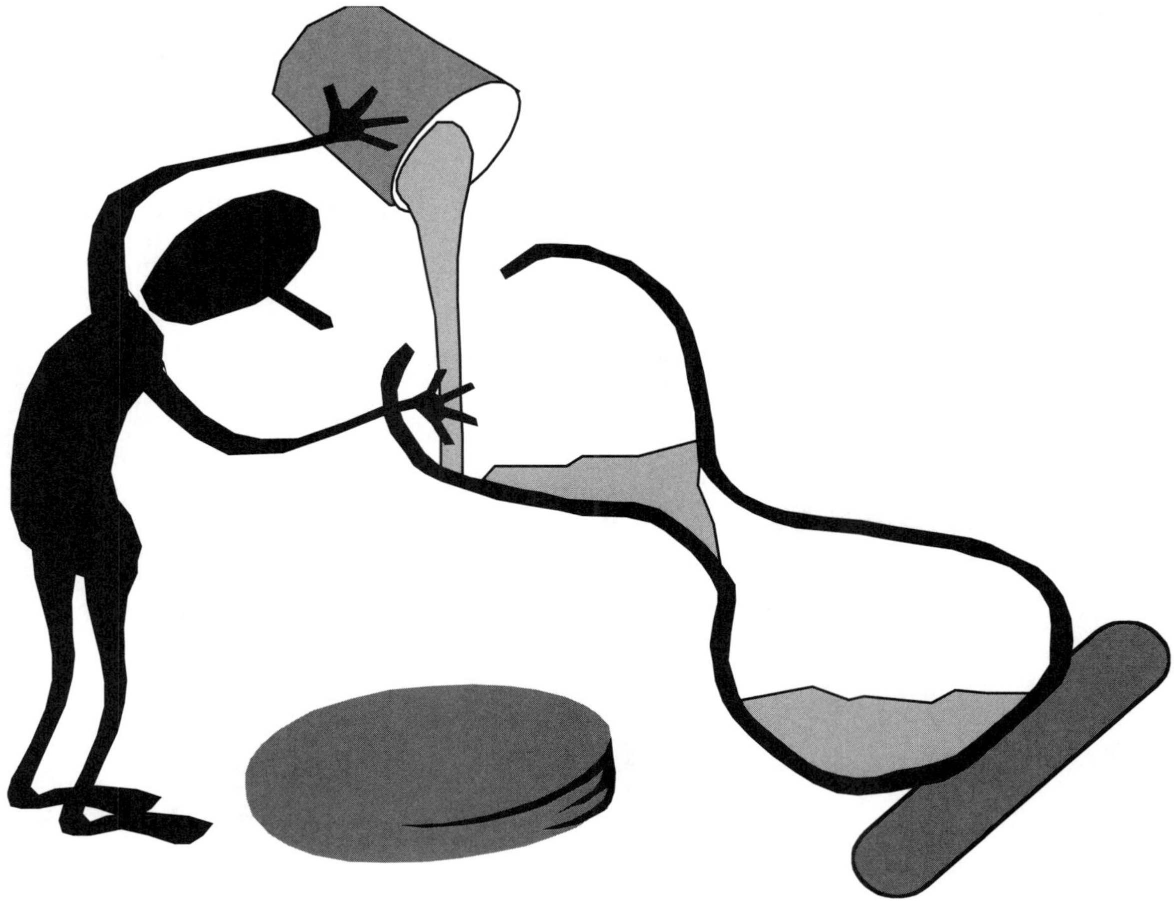

TIME MANAGEMENT

Day__________________

Group Leader Plan

Time Management Strengths and Problem Areas

I. *Objectives*: Members will be able to:
   A. Identify some of their strengths in managing their time.
   B. Identify some of their deficits in managing their time.
   C. Identify which of these deficits they would like to improve during this topic.
   D. Increase their understanding of why it is important for them to strengthen their time management skills given their dual diagnoses.

II. *Materials*: Form 2-1 and pens.

III. *Procedures*:
   A. Form 2-1, "Time Management Strengths and Problem Areas."
      1. Distribute.
      2. Have members read it aloud.
      3. Any questions?
      4. Allow time for completion.
      5. Discuss their answers.

Time Management Strengths and Problem Areas

We will be spending the next sessions talking about some of the techniques you can use to better manage your time.

Often people in recovery from drug addiction need to restructure their time to include nondrug-related activities. This means possibly developing new interests and hobbies or finding out what their community has to offer. People undergoing recovery from drug addiction often need a lot of structure in their day to help them maintain sobriety.

How you spend your time can influence how you feel about yourself. Doing activities that are productive and enjoyable help build your self-esteem. Doing activities which are nonproductive or anxiety producing can cause you to feel bad. We will spend many group sessions helping you build and stick to a schedule for yourselves that will be realistic, help you stay sober, and help you feel good about yourselves.

When people have a mental illness they often have problems with the following time management skills. Why?

1. Getting out of bed in the morning.
2. Structuring their time after the program and on weekends.
3. Following through with plans.
4. Procrastinating.
5. Prioritizing.
6. Having a daily balance of work, play, and leisure.

Keeping in mind all the time management skills we have mentioned today:

1. Which ones are you good at?

2. Which ones are you not good at?

3. Which ones would you like to work on in this group?

TIME MANAGEMENT

Day ________________

Group Leader Plan

Case Studies

I. *Objectives*: Members will be able to:
   A. Identify time management problems in the case studies.
   B. Begin to problem solve around the time management problems in the case studies.
   C. Discuss their own time management problems that are similar in nature to those in the case studies.

II. *Materials*: Form 2-2, Form 2-3, and pens.

III. *Procedures*:
   A. Form 2-2, "Case Study I."
      1. Distribute.
      2. Members read it aloud.
      3. Any questions?
      4. Allow time for completion.
      5. Discuss their answers.
         a. Case Study I answers:
            1. What has Mr. D. been doing correctly?
               - He has three months clean time.
               - He avoids drug-related people, places, things.
               - He is in a recovery program.
            2. What are Mr. D.'s problems with time management?
               - Lacks structure in his day.
               - Has not developed new hobbies or interests.
               - Does not realize that problems exist.
               - Is not aware of his feelings.
               - Has difficulty getting out of bed.
               - Is missing his program.
               - Does not ask for help.
            3. What could Mr. D. do to help himself?
               - Ask for help from his case manager.
               - Develop new hobbies and interests to include other people.
               - Socialize more while at the program.
               - Make new friends on the outside who do not use drugs or alcohol.
               - Reward himself for getting up in the morning.
               - Place his alarm clock on the other side of the room so he would have to get out of bed to turn it off.
               - Ask for a wake up call from a family member or person at residence.

- Shower before going to bed.
- Lay his clothes out the night before.
- Walk to the program with a buddy.
- Talk about increased cravings to his case manager.
- Keep a record of days he came on time and reward himself after a certain amount of times.
- Set time management goals for himself.
- Make a new schedule—cross off activities after he completes them.

4. Discuss, in depth, members' time management problems that are similar to the ones in the case study. Discuss how each member can problem solve around them.

B. Form 2-3, "Case Study II."
1. Distribute.
2. Have members read it aloud.
3. Any questions?
4. Allow time for completion.
5. Discuss their answers.
   b. Case Study II answers:
      1. Is Miss A. ready to start work tomorrow? Why? Why not?
         - No, because she has a schedule conflict; her job is 10 minutes away from school. There is not enough time to get there.
         - No, because the dog needs to be walked at 1:00, but two times out of the week Miss A. will be out.
         - No, because she needs to pick her daughter up at 3:00 P.M. on Thursdays, but she will be working until 3:00 P.M. and has a half-an-hour drive.
      2. What could Miss A. do to help herself manage time?
         - Make up a written schedule to identify problems.
         - Ask Mr. T. to walk dog (delegate work).
         - Negotiate time with her boss or her program (assert herself).
         - Consider travel time (go through the first day in her head visualizing what she needs to do, step by step).
         - Plan ahead of time.
         - Prepare a wardrobe for work.
         - Predict possible problems.
         - Eliminate problems before they happen—take control of the situation!!!
      3. Discuss, in depth, members' time management problems that are similar to the ones in the case study. Discuss how each member can work around them.

Form 2-2

Case Study I

Mr. D. is in recovery and has mental health problems. He has three months clean time. He has been able to stay away from people, places, and things related to drugs. In fact, he no longer associates with any of his old friends. He does not engage in any of his old activities because they were drug related. Mr. D. is now bored and lonely most of the time. Mr. D. finds it difficult to get out of bed in the morning and is beginning to come late or be absent from his program. Now, because he has even more time on his hands, Mr. D. is getting more cravings.

1. What has Mr. D. been doing correctly?

2. What are Mr. D.'s problems with time management?

3. What could Mr. D. do to help himself?

4. Have you ever had any of these problems?

Case Study II

Miss A. lives with her boyfriend, Mr. T. Miss A. is very excited about beginning her new volunteer job tomorrow. She will be working from 1:00–3:00 P.M. every Tuesday and Thursday. She will also continue to attend a dual diagnosis program from 9:00 A.M.–1:00 P.M. daily. Miss A.'s new job is close to her apartment, but 10 minutes from her program. Miss A. needs to walk her dog as soon as she gets home from the program because the dog is very eager to go out.

Miss A. misses her daughter, but gets to pick her up from school once a week on Thursdays at 3:00 P.M. She lives with her dad 1/2 hour away from Miss A.

1. Is Miss A. ready to start work tomorrow? Why? Why not?

2. What could Miss A. do to help herself manage her time?

3. Have you ever had any of these problems?

TIME MANAGEMENT

Day ________________

Group Leader Plan

Energy Levels*

I. *Objectives*: Members will be able to:
   A. Define "high," "medium," and "low" energy levels.
   B. Define "energy cycle."
   C. Identify their typical "high," "medium," and "low" energy times during a 24-hour day.
   D. Categorize their daily activities into "high," "medium," or "low" energy activities and state whether or not these activities match their own energy cycle. If not, what changes could be made?
   E. Learn how to be more efficient during the day.

II. *Materials*: Form 2-4, pens, and red pens.

III. *Procedures*:
   A. Form 2-4, "Energy Levels."
      1. Distribute.
      2. Define "energy levels" (the amount of energy a person has at any given time of the day) and "energy cycles" (how that energy fluctuates throughout the day).
      3. Have members plot their level of energy at any given hour of the day. Draw a curve.
      4. Discuss from the graph whether members are "morning people," "night people," or "day people."
      5. Have members add to the chart, in red pen, the times that they usually experience cravings. Is there a relationship to their level of energy?
      6. Have members list their daily activities under the correct energy level required to complete them.
   B. Do the members' daily activities fit into their natural daily energy cycles at the appropriate energy level? If not, could any helpful changes occur?
   C. Each member will identify one change in their schedule that would help them be more efficient during the day.
   D. *Homework*:
      Each member will implement the change identified and discuss the results in the next session.

*Modified with permission from Schwimmer-Stern, P. Life Skills Curriculum (unpublished master's project), 1986.

Energy Levels

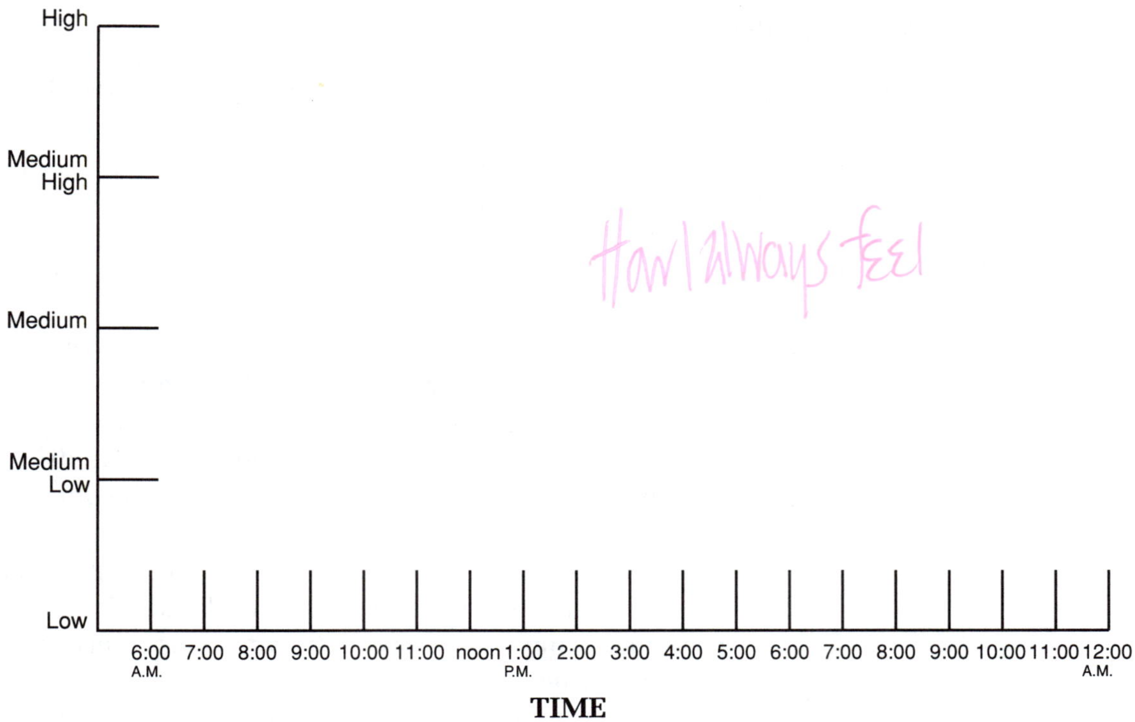

My Energy Cycle

High Energy

Times:

Activities

1)

2)

3)

4)

5)

Medium Energy

Times:

Activities

1)

2)

3)

4)

5)

Low Energy

Times:

Activities

1)

2)

3)

4)

5)

TIME MANAGEMENT

Day__________________

Group Leader Plan

What I Have to Do versus What I Like to Do (P.S. Things I Hate to Do)

I. *Objectives*: Members will be able to:
   A. Identify activities they have to do each month.
   B. Identify activities they like to do.
   C. Admit which tasks they dislike and problem solve around how to make them more enjoyable.
   D. Distinguish between the three types of activities above.
   E. Become more aware of how they spend their day.
   F. Become more aware of how they feel after their activities.
   G. Understand that they are not the only ones who have difficulty following through with things that need to be done each day.
   H. Identify which psychiatric symptoms and which symptoms of addiction interfere with each of their daily activities.
   I. Give personal examples of how their symptoms interfere with their activities.
   J. Problem solve around how to better manage their symptoms so they can perform necessary activities each day.

II. *Materials*: Table 2-1, Form 2-5, pens, blackboard, and chalk.

III. *Procedures*:
   A. Table 2-1, "Symptoms."
      1. Distribute.
      2. Have members read each symptom one at a time, discussing who has ever experienced that symptom. State that this list of symptoms should be helpful in completing the next handout.
   B. Form 2-5, "What I Have to Do versus What I Like to Do (P.S. Things I Hate to Do)."
      1. Distribute.
      2. Have members read it aloud.
      3. Any questions?
      4. Allow time for completion.
      5. Discuss their answers:
         a. Leader lists examples on the board of things the members have to do each month as members call out their answers.
         b. After a list is made, ask which symptoms interfere with each activity (writing them next to each activity).
         c. Encourage members to give personal examples of each.

d. Continue listing activities that members like to do plus interfering symptoms, then things they hate to do and what would make those things more enjoyable.
e. Incorporate discrepancies in how often things are done and how often members do or would like to do them with the symptoms that interfere with each activity.
f. Promote problem solving around how to better manage their symptoms in order to complete necessary tasks.

Table 2-1 Symptoms

Some Symptoms of Mental Illness
Hearing voices that are not really there (auditory hallucinations)
Seeing things that are not really there (visual hallucinations)
Believing things that are not really true (delusions)
Difficulty getting up in the morning
Being unmotivated
Low energy
Having intrusive thoughts
Difficulty making decisions
Problems adjusting to change
Not getting pleasure out of things
Believing that people are out to get you

Some Symptoms of Addiction
Cravings
Anxiety
Low self-esteem
Feeling different from other people
Poor social boundaries
Being passive or aggressive, but not assertive
Difficulty accepting responsibility
Fear of failure
Fear of success
Fear of change
Feeling bored, empty, hopeless, numb, angry, guilty, or depressed
Denial
Poor health

What I Have to Do versus What I Like to Do
(P.S. Things I Hate to Do)

Things I Have to Do Every Month	*How Often Do They Need to Be Done?*	*How Often Do I Do Them?*	*Symptoms That Interfere*
1.			
2.			
3.			
4.			
5.			
6.			
7.			
8.			
9.			
10.			

Things I Like to Do	*How Often Do I Do Them?*	*How Often Would I Like to Do Them?*	*Symptoms That Interfere*
1.			
2.			
3.			
4.			
5.			
6.			
7.			
8.			
9.			
10.			

Things I Hate to Do	*What Could Make Them More Enjoyable?*
1.	
2.	
3.	
4.	
5.	
6.	
7.	
8.	
9.	
10.	

TIME MANAGEMENT

Day ____________________

Group Leader Plan

How I Currently Spend My Time*

I. *Objectives*: Members will be able to:
   A. Record how they currently spend their time in a typical weekday and weekend day.
   B. Record how they feel during each daily activity.
   C. Gain an overall view of how their time is structured.
   D. State what they like and dislike about their schedules.
   E. State what changes they would like to make in their schedules for the future.

II. *Materials*: Form 2-6 and pens.

III. *Procedures*:
   A. Form 2-6, "How I Currently Spend My Time."
      1. Distribute.
      2. Have members read it aloud.
      3. Explain the objectives of the form (A–E above).
      4. Any questions?
      5. Allow time for completion.
      6. Discuss their answers.
      7. Ask, "What do you like and dislike about your current schedule?"
      8. Ask, "What changes in your schedule would you like to make in the future?"
      9. Discuss how their feelings can be related to their activities or vice versa.

*Modified with permission from Schwimmer-Stern, P. Life Skills Curriculum (unpublished master's project), 1986.

How I Currently Spend My Time

Please fill in, by the hour, what a typical weekday and weekend day were like in your life last week. Next to each activity, please state how you felt when you did it.

Weekday	*How I Felt*
6:00 A.M.	
7:00 A.M.	
8:00 A.M.	
9:00 A.M.	
10:00 A.M.	
11:00 A.M.	
12:00 P.M.	
1:00 P.M.	
2:00 P.M.	
3:00 P.M.	
4:00 P.M.	
5:00 P.M.	
6:00 P.M.	
7:00 P.M.	
8:00 P.M.	
9:00 P.M.	
10:00 P.M.	
11:00 P.M.	
12:00 A.M.	
1:00 A.M.	
2:00 A.M.	
3:00 A.M.	
4:00 A.M.	
5:00 A.M.	

Form 2-6 (*continued*)

Weekend Day	*How I Felt*
6:00 A.M.	
7:00 A.M.	
8:00 A.M.	
9:00 A.M.	
10:00 A.M.	
11:00 A.M.	
12:00 P.M.	
1:00 P.M.	
2:00 P.M.	
3:00 P.M.	
4:00 P.M.	
5:00 P.M.	
6:00 P.M.	
7:00 P.M.	
8:00 P.M.	
9:00 P.M.	
10:00 P.M.	
11:00 P.M.	
12:00 A.M.	
1:00 A.M.	
2:00 A.M.	
3:00 A.M.	
4:00 A.M.	
5:00 A.M.	

TIME MANAGEMENT

Day__________________

Group Leader

The Need for Structure to Stay Clean

I. *Objectives*: Members will be able to:
   A. Define what is meant by "structure."
   B. Verbalize how structure can help them stay clean.
   C. Explain how the lack of structure can cause a relapse.
   D. Explain how time management can be used to reduce stress.
   E. Make a change in their schedule so that their days may have more structure through the use of short-term goals.

II. *Materials*: None.

III. *Procedures*:
   A. Discuss the following topics:
      1. Define what is meant by "structured" and "unstructured."
      2. Ask members to give examples of times of the day that they have picked up in the past. Were they during unstructured times?
      3. When do members most frequently get cravings? During structured or unstructured times?
      4. Discuss the law of inertia—how the world, if left alone tends toward chaos and unraveling (for example, a grassy area becomes a field of overgrown weeds).
         Discuss how drugs, alcohol, and mental illness can cause one's life to become unmanageable and unstructured (for example, a clean apartment becomes a dirty apartment which leads to eviction). Discuss how members must put constant effort into maintaining and bettering their lives using structure.
      5. Discuss concrete examples of how people's weekdays are different from their weekends (structured time vs. unstructured time).
      6. Discuss how the key to structuring their time is through setting short-term, daily, or weekly goals.
      7. Discuss how structuring their time can reduce anxiety and inertia.
   B. *Homework*:
      Members each pick one way (activity) to add more structure to their schedule. Share it at the end of the group. For homework, encourage members to do that activity during an unstructured part of their day. Have them report their progress in the next session.

TIME MANAGEMENT

Day__________________

Group Leader

Activity Analysis

I. *Objectives*: Members will be able to:
   A. Analyze a current activity they enjoy.
   B. Select alcohol and drug free activities that are realistic, meet their needs, and will help maintain sobriety.
   C. Commit to adding one new activity to their lives.

II. *Materials*: Form 2-7 (two for each member), pens, blackboard, and chalk.

III. *Procedures*:
   A. Form 2-7, "Activity Analysis."
      1. Group leader example of an activity analysis:
         a. Distribute Form 2-7, "Activity Analysis."
         b. Go through an activity of your choice, answering all the questions about it.
         c. Have members fill in your answers.
         d. For each question that you answered "yes" to, put a "✓" under "important" if it is important to you. Leave it blank if it is not important to you.
         e. Give an example of another activity that would meet your needs, that is, have the same "important" characteristics.
         f. You have just taught the members how to do an activity analysis.
      2. Members' activity analysis:
         a. Distribute Form 2-7, "Activity Analysis," again.
         b. Ask members to pick a different activity they enjoy doing and fill out the Activity Analysis as you just did, but with their activity.
         c. Any questions?
         d. Allow time for completion.
         e. Discuss their answers.
   B. *Homework*:
      The homework assignment is listed at the end of Form 2-7, "Activity Analysis." Have members read it aloud and complete it before the next session. Discuss their answers in the next session.

Activity Analysis

Identify Activity____

Characteristics	*Yes*	*No*	*Important*
1. Is it social?			
2. Does it require rules?			
3. Is it expensive?			
4. Can it be done anytime?			
5. Can it be done anywhere?			
6. Does it involve a lot of skill?			
7. Is it pleasurable?			
8. Is it a high energy activity?			
9. Is it easy to learn?			
10. Can you do it alone?			
11. Does it require equipment?			
12. Is it competitive?			

What other activities have similar characteristics to the ones you said were important to you?

Of these, pick one that you would like to start in the near future. List it below.

Homework: Find out one new thing about this activity that you did not previously know. Discuss it in the next group session.

TIME MANAGEMENT

Day__________________

Group Leader Plan

Delegating Work

I. *Objectives*: Members will be able to:
   A. Identify why it is difficult for them to ask for help.
   B. State how delegating work can be a useful time management technique.
   C. Identify who in their own lives they could delegate work to.
   D. Identify how other people in their lives could help them.

II. *Materials*: Form 2-8 and pens.

III. *Procedures*:
   A. Form 2-8, "Delegating Work."
      1. Distribute.
      2. Have members read it aloud.
      3. Any questions?
      4. Allow time for completion.
      5. Discuss their answers, emphasizing the objectives above.
   B. *Homework*:
      1. Have members read the assignment on the bottom of the handout aloud.
      2. Have them state who they will ask for help and what kind of help they will ask for by next session.
      3. Follow-up at the beginning of the next session.

Delegating Work

One of the ways we can better manage our time is by asking others for assistance or delegating work. This works especially well if we have too many things to do or if we do not have the resources it takes to get something done.

Yet, a lot of people have difficulty asking for help. Maybe they are not assertive enough. They may feel guilty. They may be afraid of rejection. They may be disorganized. Or, for some, asking for help means giving up some control and swallowing some pride.

Sound familiar? Is it hard for you to ask for help? Why?

The following are examples of delegating work:

1. I would like my daughter to share in the housework.
2. I would like my neighbor to feed my cat when I am ill.
3. I would like my father to respect my sobriety and stop asking me if I want a drink every time I visit him.

Now, you delegate work by filling in the blanks below:

1. I would like my ____________________ to ______________________________________

   ____.

2. I would like my ____________________ to ______________________________________

   ____.

3. I would like my ____________________ to ______________________________________

   ____.

Homework: Choose one person above and ask that person to help you in the way you have described. Tell us how it went next session.

TIME MANAGEMENT

Day ________________

Group Leader Plan

Leisure Community Resources

I. *Objectives*: Members will be able to:
   A. Look up addresses and phone numbers of community leisure resources.
   B. Be more aware of leisure activities.
   C. Teach and inform others of their knowledge of leisure community resources and upcoming events of interest.
   D. Learn different resources to plan leisure time.

II. *Materials*: Form 2-9, Form 2-10, and pens.

III. *Procedures*:
   A. Form 2-9, "Leisure Community Resources."
      1. Distribute.
      2. Have members read it aloud.
      3. Any questions?
      4. Members can work as a group, individually, or in pairs to complete as many of the questions as possible. They can use the phone book or any other resource guide you provide.
      5. Any questions that members cannot complete in the group are divided up and chosen for homework.
   B. Form 2-10, "Homework."
      1. Distribute.
      2. Have members read it aloud.
      3. Any questions?
      4. Members should commit to one assignment before the group ends.
      5. For the following session please bring in as many materials as you can from the homework assignment to supplement what the members bring in.
      6. Review what they bring in next session.

Leisure Community Resources

Please record the name and address of the following community resources nearest your home.

1. Your clinic's address:
2. Your clinic's phone number:
3. 12-step meeting:
4. Library:
5. What else besides books does this library offer?
6. Place of worship:
7. What other services does this place of worship offer?
8. Leisure information center:
9. Museum:
10. Theater:
11. Parks:
12. What other activities does this park sponsor?

List all the different resources you could use to plan your leisure time:

1.	8.
2.	9.
3.	10.
4.	11.
5.	12.
6.	13.
7.	14.

Form 2-10

Homework

Choose one of the following and complete it before next session. You can work in pairs.

1. Bring in a pamphlet from the nearest place of worship of your faith that describes some of the other activities this congregation has to offer.
2. Bring in a pamphlet from the nearest library that describes some of the activities the library has to offer.
3. Bring in a pamphlet from the nearest museum stating the hours of operation and the fees.
4. Bring in a schedule of movies from a theater.
5. Bring in a list of 12-step meetings in your neighborhood that states the time and place of each meeting offered.
6. Bring in a newspaper and show the group how to find the leisure section and what different things appear there.
7. Inform the group of an upcoming event in your neighborhood. Be specific—time, place, cost, and so on.
8. Bring in a subway map or bus map and state one place you would visit using public transportation.
9. Bring in a pamphlet from a leisure information center on activities in your neighborhood.

TIME MANAGEMENT

Day__________________

Group Leader Plan

Weekend Planning

I. *Objectives*: Members will be able to:
   A. Restructure their weekends to better meet their needs.
   B. Follow through with the activities planned and report their progress in the next session.
II. *Materials*: Form 2-11 and pens.
III. *Procedures*:
   A. Form 2-11, "Weekend Planning."
      1. Distribute.
      2. Have members read it aloud.
      3. Any questions?
      4. Allow time for completion.
      5. Discuss their answers.
      6. Review their progress after the weekend in the next session.
   B. *Homework*:
      Each member should follow through with his or her goal related to weekend planning and discuss it next session.

Form 2-11

Weekend Planning

I am going to make the following plans for this weekend

New activity to add:

Why did I choose this new activity?

Steps I need to take in order to plan for the new activity:

1.

2.

3.

4.

Where will the new activity fit in my existing weekend schedule?

TIME MANAGEMENT

Day___________________

Group Leader Plan

Revising My Weekly Schedule*

I. *Objectives*: Members will be able to:
   A. Review past material and use it to revise their schedules so that they will:
      1. Have a better daily balance of work, play, and leisure.
      2. Engage in more purposeful activities.
      3. Better manage psychiatric symptoms.
      4. Avoid acting on drug cravings and triggers.
      5. Broaden their leisure interests.
      6. Increase their social contacts.
      7. Better structure their time.
      8. Feel better about themselves.
      9. Plan and carry out their goals.

II. *Materials*: Form 2-12, Form 2-13, and pens.

III. *Procedures*:
   A. Form 2-12, "Revising My Weekly Schedule," and Form 2-13, "Revised Schedule."
      1. Distribute.
      2. Have members read it aloud.
      3. Any questions?
      4. Allow time for completion.
      5. Review.
   B. *Homework*:
      Members are to follow their schedules, checking off each activity they completed. When reporting this progress at the next session, they are to state why they could not complete an activity that was difficult for them.

*Modified with permission from Schwimmer-Stern, P. Life Skills Curriculum (unpublished master's project), 1986.

Revising My Weekly Schedule

Over the last few sessions, you were able to add more structured, planned activities to your weekends. These additional activities helped to:

1. Better structure your time.
2. Encourage you to engage in more purposeful activities.
3. Learn new things.
4. See that you can plan and carry out goals.
5. Increase your social network.
6. Avoid cravings and triggers.
7. Broaden your leisure interests.

For the next few sessions, you are going to rewrite your weekly schedules. You may add additional meetings or activities to provide more structure. You may switch activities around to fit your energy levels. Whatever changes you make, make them realistic. You will be asked to follow your schedule as closely as possible and report on your progress next session.

Fill in your revised schedule on the following page. Incorporate all the things that you have learned about yourself in time management. How is this schedule different from your usual schedule?

Homework: Follow your schedule. Put an "X" through each activity you followed through with. If you are unable to follow through with the activity, state why on the back of your schedule.

Revised Schedule

Day **Name:** ____________________

	8:00 A.M.	9:00	10:00	11:00	12:00 P.M.	1:00	2:00	3:00	4:00
Monday									
Tuesday									
Wednesday									
Thursday									
Friday									
Saturday									
Sunday									

Form 2-13 (*continued*)

Revised Schedule

Evening

Name: ______________________

	5:00 P.M.	6:00	7:00	8:00	9:00	10:00	11:00	12:00 A.M.
Monday								
Tuesday								
Wednesday								
Thursday								
Friday								
Saturday								
Sunday								

TIME MANAGEMENT

Day ____________________

Group Leader Plan

Sticking to a New Schedule

I. *Objectives*: Members will be able to:
   A. Report which scheduled activity they were able to follow.
   B. Report which scheduled activity they were not able to complete, and what made it difficult to complete it.
   C. Problem solve around how they can stick to their schedules more effectively using previously learned time management techniques.
   D. Continue to revise their schedules to better meet their goals.

II. *Materials*: Previous handout Form 2-13, "Revised Schedule," and pens.

III. *Procedures*:
   A. Review Form 2-13, "Revised Schedule."
      1. Have members state which activities they completed. Give them positive reinforcement for their achievements.
      2. Have members state which activities they did not complete and why.
      3. Have each member problem solve around how to make it easier to perform these uncompleted activities or how to modify them if need be.
      4. Have members give each other feedback on how to make it easier to follow their new schedule.
   B. *Homework*:
      Each member tries again to follow their revised schedule and reports their progress in the following session.

TIME MANAGEMENT

Day __________________

Group Leader Plan

Rewarding Myself*

I. *Objectives*: Members will be able to:
   A. Understand the importance of recognition in motivation and self-esteem.
   B. Be able to reward themselves.
   C. Be able to accept praise from others.

II. *Materials*: Form 2-14 and pens.

III. *Procedures*:
   A. Define rewards.
   B. Discuss why and how daily rewards are important.
   C. Form 2-14, "Rewarding Myself."
      1. Distribute.
      2. Have members read it aloud.
      3. Any questions?
      4. Allow time for completion.
      5. Discuss their answers.
   D. *Homework*:
      Members will follow through with rewarding themselves as they defined in their handouts.

*Modified with permission from Korb, K. L., Azok, S., and Leutenberg E. A. *Life Management Skills III.* Beachwood, OH: Wellness Reproductions, Inc., 1994, p. 24.

Rewarding Myself

I would like to reward myself when I . . .	*These are a few of my favorite rewards . . .*
1.	1.
2.	2.
3.	3.
4.	4.
5.	5.
6.	6.
7.	7.
8.	8.

Homework: Between now and next session, I will follow through with rewarding myself as I have described above.

TIME MANAGEMENT

Day ________________

Group Leader Plan

Getting Up in the Morning

I. *Objectives*: Members will be able to:
   A. Problem solve around how to make it easier to get up in the morning.
   B. Use at least one of these techniques so they can make it to an appointment on time.

II. *Materials*: Form 2-15 and pens.

III. *Procedures*:
   A. Form 2-15, "Getting Up in the Morning."
      1. Distribute.
      2. Have members read it aloud.
      3. Any questions?
      4. Allow time for completion.
      5. Discuss their answers. Help members problem solve with the following solutions:
         a. Alarm clock.
         b. Wake up call.
         c. Get a healthy breakfast.
         d. Shower after awakening.
         e. Shower the night before.
         f. Lay out clothes before going to bed.
         g. Set alarm across the room.
         h. Think ahead about the consequences of being late.
         i. Set goals with therapist.
         j. No caffeine the night before.
         k. Go to sleep early enough.
         l. Wake up at the same time every morning.
         m. Go to bed at the same time every night.
         n. Avoid sleeping during the day.
         o. Do not eat before going to bed.
         p. Reward yourself.
         q. Plan your day the night before.
         r. Start your day with something you look forward to doing.
         s. Get a pet that will wake you up in the morning: cat, dog, or bird.
         t. Take an invigorating shower.
         u. Exercise.
         v. Sleep with the curtains open so sun can come in.
         w. Stop using drugs and alcohol.

B. *Homework*:
Members will choose one or two techniques from their lists that they will try between now and next session to improve their ability to wake up in the morning. Members will report their progress in the following session.

Form 2-15

Getting Up in the Morning

Oh, how I hate to get up in the morning . . . ZZZZZZZZZZZZZZZ

List all the ways you could think of to help someone get up in the morning.

Homework: Choose one method that you listed above and use it daily to improve your ability to start your day on time.

3 Stress Management for Recovery

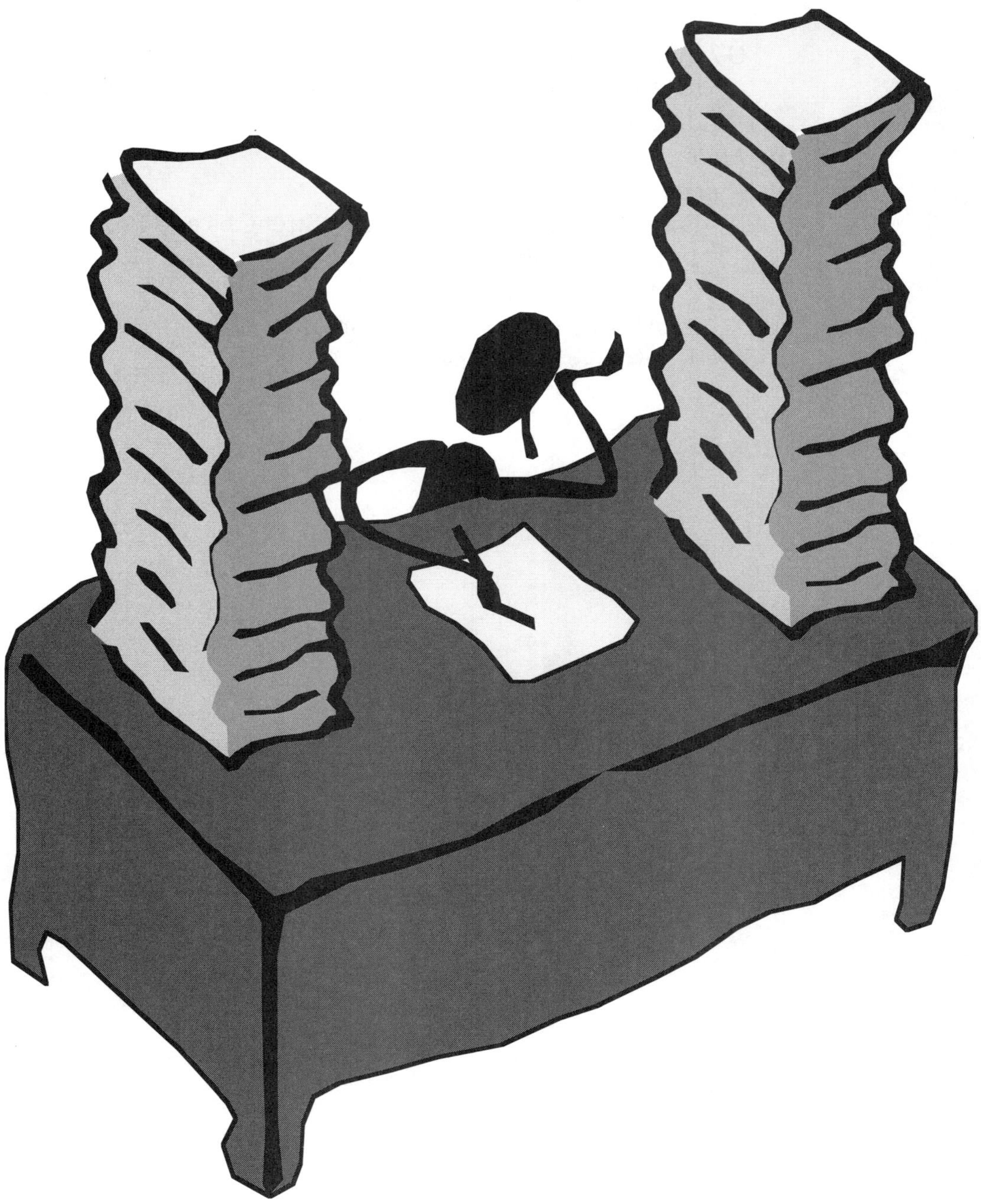

STRESS MANAGEMENT

Day__________________

Group Leader Plan

Stress Management Strengths and Problem Areas

I. *Objectives*: All members will be able to:
   A. Identify some of their strengths in managing stress.
   B. Identify some of their deficits in managing stress.
   C. Identify which of these deficits they will work on improving during this group.
   D. Increase their understanding of why it is important for them to strengthen their stress management skills given their dual diagnoses.

II. *Materials*: Form 3-1 and pens.

III. *Procedures*:
   A. Form 3-1, "Stress Management Strengths and Problem Areas."
      1. Have members read it aloud.
      2. Any questions?
      3. Allow time for completion.
      4. Discuss their answers.

Stress Management Strengths and Problem Areas

We will be spending the next sessions on learning and practicing stress management techniques. This way you can do them on your own whenever you need to.

Everyone experiences stress at some time or another. You cannot change all of the things that cause you stress, but you can learn how to better handle stressful situations while remaining clean and sober. You may have clean time, but it is often a stressful situation that can trigger a relapse. Developing specific stress management techniques can help prevent relapse and help you make a smoother transition to the community when you are ready to move on.

Some stress management techniques that help stop stress from getting to the point where you pick up are:

1. Keeping stress management diaries.
2. Anger management.
3. Problem solving.
4. Goal setting.
5. Assertiveness training.

How do these techniques help?

When people have mental health problems they often have problems with the following stress management skills:

1. Relaxation.
2. Proper nutrition.
3. Exercise.
4. Identifying stressful situations.

Why do you think these are problems?

Keeping in mind all the stress management skills we have mentioned today:

1. Which ones are you good at?

2. Which ones are you *not* good at?

3. Which ones would you like to work on in this group?

STRESS MANAGEMENT

Day__________________

Group Leader Plan

How Stressed Am I?

I. *Objectives*: Members will be able to:
   A. Report their current symptoms of stress.
   B. Determine their current level of stress.
II. *Materials*: Form 3-2 and pens.
III. *Procedures*:
   A. Form 3-2, "How Stressed Am I?"
      1. Give verbal directions—members should check "yes" if the statement pertains to them and "no" if it is not true of them at this time.
      2. Have members read form aloud.
      3. Any questions?
      4. Allow time for completion.
      5. Discuss their answers.
      6. Calculate their level of stress.
         a. Total the number of "yes" answers. This is their score.
         b. If their score falls between:
            0–2 then they are experiencing low levels of stress.
            3–4 then they are experiencing moderate levels of stress.
            5 + then they are experiencing high levels of stress.
      7. Give members feedback about their scores.

How Stressed Am I?

	Check Below Yes	No
My neck and back are often sore.		
I get many headaches.		
My stomach feels like it is in knots at times.		
I feel overwhelmed easily.		
I get irritable and cranky.		
I have difficulty getting out of my bed in the morning to face the day.		
Being around people makes me anxious.		
I have difficulty sleeping at night.		
My thoughts race in my head.		
I worry a lot.		
I have had a recent death of someone close to me.		
Someone in my family is sick.		
I am unhappy with where I live.		
I do not have any friends.		
I am lonely most of the time.		
I just started a new job or volunteer work.		
I moved within this last year.		

Total # of "yes" answers __________

This puts me in the ______________________ stress category.
(High, Moderate, Low)

STRESS MANAGEMENT

Day ________________

Group Plan Leader

Signs of Stress

I. *Objectives*: Members will be able to:
   A. Describe how they react to stress.
   B. Identify their first warning sign of stress.
   C. Practice stopping a stressful activity at the first warning sign of stress.
   D. Begin to redirect their behavior as a way to manage this stress before it becomes overwhelming and unmanageable.

II. *Materials*: Form 3-3, blackboard, chalk, and pens.

III. *Procedures*:
   A. Form 3-3, "Signs of Stress."
      1. Have members read it aloud.
      2. Any questions?
      3. Allow time for completion.
      4. Discuss their answers. As members call out their stress signals list them on the board.
   B. *Homework*:
      Have members look for their first warning sign of stress in their daily lives. When they notice their sign they should stop and manage their stress. Members will report their progress next session.

Form 3-3

Signs of Stress

List below all the ways you react to stress.

Which of these is the first reaction that happens?

____

____

____

____

This is your first warning sign that you are becoming stressed. When you feel this, you need to STOP and MANAGE YOUR STRESS.

STRESS MANAGEMENT

Day________________

Group Leader Plan

Environmental Stressors

I. *Objectives*: Members will be able to:
   A. Define "environmental stressors."
   B. Identify their environmental stressors.
   C. Chart the severity of each of these stressors.
   D. Understand that stress rises and falls in a bell-shaped curve.
   E. Understand that they can learn to manage their stress before it reaches a peak, and that stress will eventually decrease again.
   F. Realize that they cannot always change the stressors in their environment, but they can change the way they cope with these stressors by learning and practicing new, healthy, stress-management techniques that work for them.
   G. Learn that in small amounts stress can be motivating and helpful.

II. *Materials*: Form 3-4, Group Leader Plan, "Completed Bell-Shaped Curve," blackboard, chalk, and pens.

III. *Procedures*:
   A. Define "environmental stressors"—challenging, frustrating, or overwhelming events such as attending an Alcoholics Anonymous meeting for the first time or setting up discharge plans.
   B. Identify environmental stressors and their severity.
      1. Distribute Form 3-4, "Environmental Stressors."
      2. Draw a bell-shaped curve on the blackboard as in Form 3-4, "Environmental Stressors." Explain aspects of the bell-shaped curve: time, amount of stress, the curve.
      3. Ask clients to give specific examples of their environmental stressors and how severe they are (0–100%). Record them on a board in the appropriate portion of the bell curve with a dot and a label.
      4. At the same time, have clients fill in their own bell-shaped curves with stressors as they call them out to the group leader.
      5. Fill in the whole bell shape with identified stressors from all group members in this fashion. (For steps 2–4, see Group Leader Plan, "Completed Bell-Shaped Curve.")
   C. Explain how stress rises and falls in a bell-shaped curve, instead of coming on suddenly out of nowhere.
   D. Explain that members can learn to stop the stress before it reaches the peak and becomes overwhelming. (Draw railroad tracks in curve at the 50% mark.)

E. Emphasize that there will always be environmental stress, but members can learn how to better cope with it instead of using drugs and alcohol.
F. Discuss that this group will teach them new, healthy, stress-management techniques which they will practice at home.

Form 3-4

Environmental Stressors

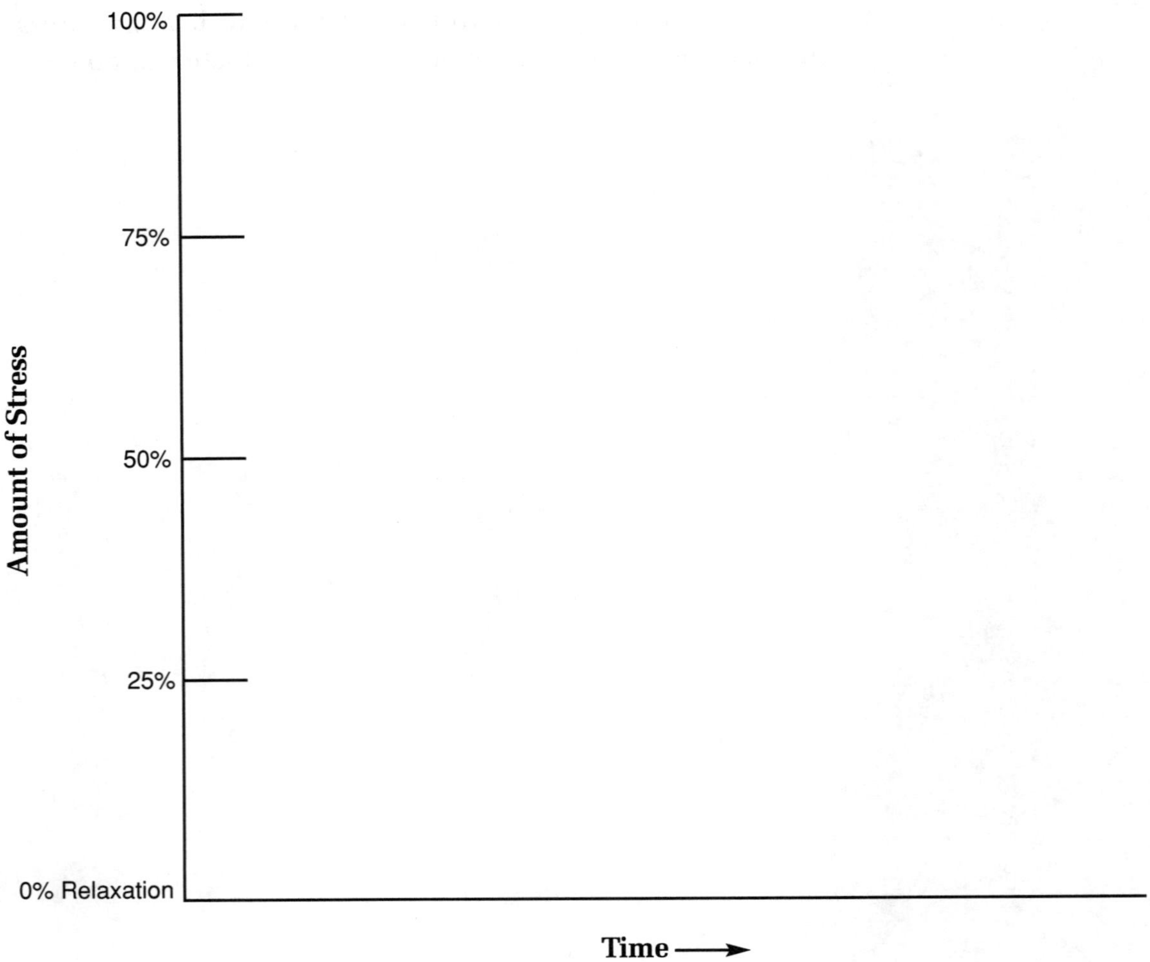

STRESS MANAGEMENT

Day ____________________

Group Leader Plan

Completed Bell-Shaped Curve (Example)

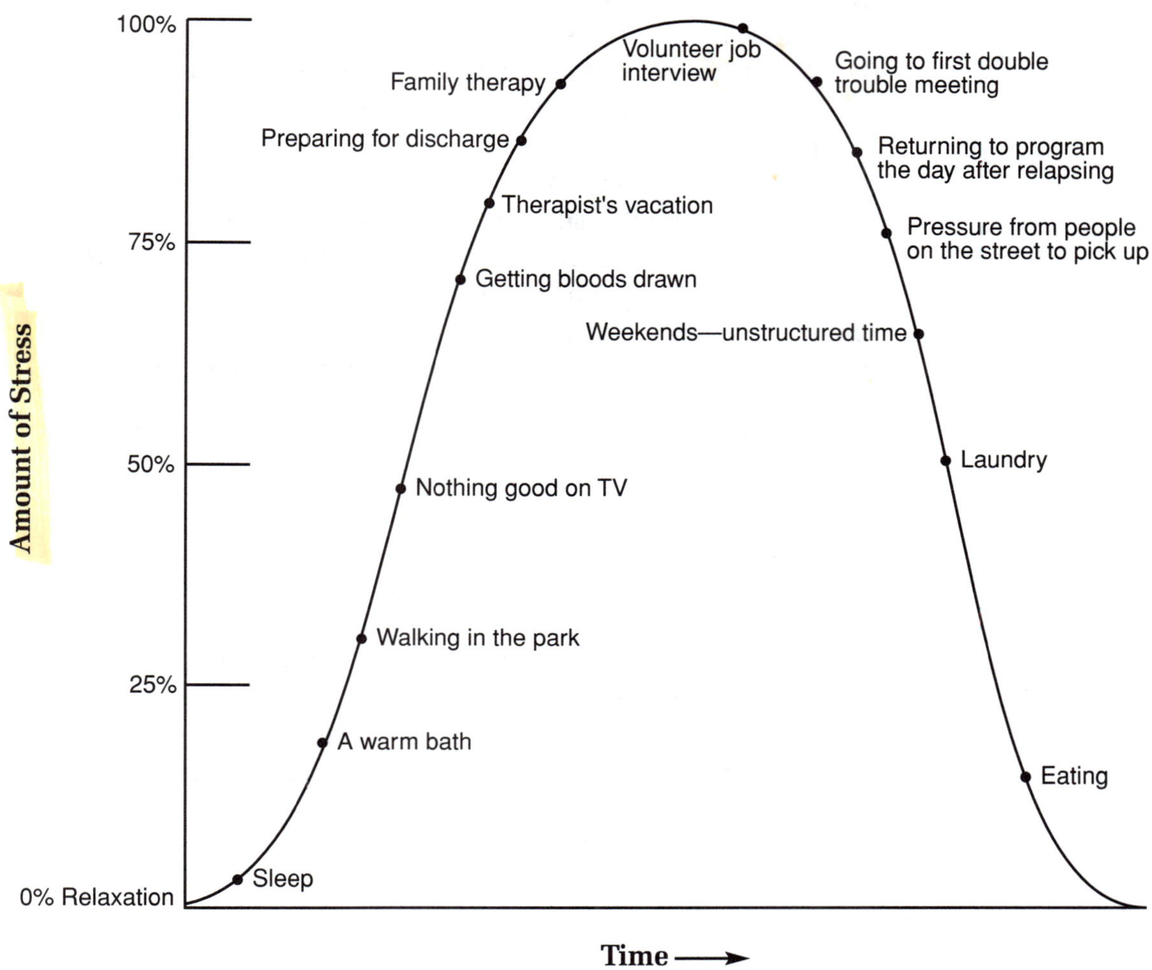

STRESS MANAGEMENT

Day____________________

Group Leader Plan

Healthy and Unhealthy Ways to Deal with Stress

I. *Objectives*: Members will be able to:
   A. List unhealthy ways to deal with stress.
   B. Identify current unhealthy ways that they deal with stress.
   C. Identify past unhealthy methods for dealing with their stress.
   D. List healthy ways to deal with stress.
   E. Identify current healthy ways that they deal with stress.
   F. Identify past healthy methods for dealing with their stress.

II. *Materials*: Form 3-5, blackboard, and pens.

III. *Procedures*:
   A. Form 3-5, "Healthy and Unhealthy Ways to Deal with Stress."
      1. Distribute.
      2. Have members read it aloud.
      3. Any questions?
      4. Have members fill out both columns.
      5. Have members call out their answers for each column as you write them on the board.
      6. Ask members to put an "*" next to the healthy and unhealthy ways that they *currently* use.
      7. Ask clients to put a "✓" next to the healthy and unhealthy ways that they have managed stress in the *past*.
      8. Discuss examples from each member.

Healthy and Unhealthy Ways to Deal with Stress

Healthy	*Unhealthy*

STRESS MANAGEMENT

Day ____________________

Group Leader Plan

Stress Management Journal

I. *Objectives*: Members will be able to:
   A. Identify one stressful event each day for a week.
   B. Describe their resultant behavior.
   C. State a new stress management technique that they could have used in that situation.
   D. Become more aware of their daily stressors.
   E. Document the cause and effect relationship that stress has on their behavior.
   F. Record how they are currently dealing with stress.

II. *Materials*: Form 3-6 and pens.

III. *Procedures*:
   A. Form 3-6, "Stress Management Journal."
      1. Distribute.
      2. Have members read it aloud.
      3. Any questions?
      4. Have members record one stressful event from today. Have them record what they did and list a new stress management technique that they could try in that situation.
      5. Discuss everyone's answers, encouraging feedback from members around new stress management techniques.
   B. *Homework*:
      Members will make daily entries until their Stress Management Journals are complete for one week. Go over their answers in the next session. Encourage members to continue these journals as one form of stress management.

Form 3-6

Stress Management Journal*

	Stressful Event	*How I Reacted*	*New Stress Management Techniques I Could Try*
Monday			
Tuesday			
Wednesday			
Thursday			
Friday			
Saturday			
Sunday			

*Modified from: Field, F. *Guide to Stress without Distress.*

STRESS MANAGEMENT

Day__________________

Group Leader Plan

Many Ways to Manage Stress and Prevent a Relapse

I. *Objectives*: Members will be able to:
   A. Learn new stress management techniques.
   B. Choose stress management techniques that would be appropriate for them to try in their own daily lives to aid in recovery.
   C. Discuss which techniques have worked or not worked for them in the past.
   D. Choose one stress management technique from a list that they have never tried before, and do it between now and the next session. Members will report their progress next session.

II. *Materials*: Form 3-7 and pens.

III. *Procedures*:
   A. Form 3-7, "Many Ways to Manage Stress and Prevent a Relapse."
      1. Distribute.
      2. Have each member read aloud one stress management technique at a time with discussion in between.
      3. Have members define each technique.
      4. Discuss if members agree or disagree whether each is a good way to manage stress, giving examples from their life experiences.
   B. *Homework*:
      Have each member choose one new technique from the list that they have never tried before and circle it on their forms. Members should practice that technique daily until next session, then report their progress. This assignment may be repeated for several sessions.

Many Ways to Manage Stress and Prevent a Relapse

Exercise Daily

Identify Your Triggers

Manage Your Time

Stay Away from People, Places, and Things

Prioritize Your Duties

Manage Your Cravings

Problem Solve

Attend Double Trouble Meetings

Assert Yourself

Forgive Yourself

Stop Thinking Negative Thoughts

Surrender to Your Higher Power

Have a Daily Balance of Work, Play, and Leisure

Make a Personal Inventory

Develop Drug/Alcohol Free Hobbies

Be More Aware of Your Denial

Take a Walk

Do Not Wait for Someone Else to Help You

Make Decisions

Learn from Your Relapses

Be More Independent

Identify Your Risky Behaviors

Love Yourself

Develop Sobriety

Love Someone Else

Accept Rehabilitation Treatment or Detoxification if Needed

Be Around Animals

Sing

Form 3-7 (*continued*)

Express Your Feelings

Talk About Your Problems

Manage Your Anger

Live in the Here and Now, Not in the Past or the Future

Take Breaks

Plan Ahead for Leisure Activities

Eat Properly and Regularly

Get Enough Sleep

Do Stretching Exercises

Yoga

Deep Breathing

Listen to Music

Be with People Who Give You Positive Feelings

Make Lists of Things to Do

Count to Ten and Walk Away from Stress

Predict Stressful Situations

Stop Unwanted Thoughts

Realize Your Strengths

Realize Your Limits

Be Able to Say "No"

Identify What You Want Out of Life

Take One Step at a Time

Be in a Drug/Alcohol Free Environment

Use Humor

Take One Day at a Time

Keep a Daily Stress Journal

Do Something for Yourself Daily

Reward Yourself

Delegate Work

Meditate

Pursue a Sport

Read the Comics

Look Nice

Sit in the Sun

Tell Jokes

Collect Something

Stop Making Excuses

Move Forward—Follow through with Short-Term Goals

Budget or Save Your Money

Remember Beautiful Scenery

Eliminate Caffeine from Your Diet

Eliminate Sugar from Your Diet

Eliminate Salt from Your Diet

Find a Place You Can Relax

Eat Tasty Foods

Develop a Support Network

Stay Clean

Ask for Clarification if You Do Not Understand Something

Set Limits for Yourself

Mental Imagery

Avoid Stressful Situations

Ask for Help

Identify Your Feelings

Know Your Symptoms of Stress

Participate in Life

Take Care of Yourself

Set Aside Time for Fun

View Stress Management Videos

Listen to Stress Management Tapes

Swim

Paint

STRESS MANAGEMENT

Day __________________

Group Leader Plan

Relaxation Skills

I. *Objectives*: Members will be able to:
   A. Rid themselves of extraneous thoughts.
   B. Practice sitting quietly.
   C. Focus their attention on their breathing.
   D. Engage in deep breathing exercises.
   E. Perform guided tension release exercises.
   F. Discuss what differences they notice in themselves after having performed the exercises above.
   G. State when and where they could perform these stress management techniques at home.
   H. Practice these techniques at home and report their progress.
   I. State how these techniques aid in managing stress and in their recovery.

II. *Materials*: A large, quiet, dark room with floor space; mats; relaxing music; comfortable, loose fitting clothes; matches and candles.

III. *Procedures*:
   A. Ask if any members have ever done deep breathing exercises, yoga, meditation, visual imagery, or tension-release exercises. Ask them to explain.
   B. Fill in any information regarding the above that the members did not define.
   C. Set up the room by spreading out the mats, explaining the need for a low stimulus environment: dim, quiet, and spacious.
   D. Explain what the deep breathing exercise entails: how long the exercise will last, that members will be lying down on mats, with their eyes closed, in a comfortable position, that they will concentrate on your voice and your instructions and perform the deep breathing exercises as you describe. Emphasize that this is not hypnosis. The exercise is meant to be relaxing, so if a member begins to feel uncomfortable and cannot refocus, they can listen in a sitting position or leave the group.
   E. Deep breathing exercise.
      1. Have clients lay down on mats.
      2. Turn lights off, close shades and doors.
      3. Put on low, relaxing background music.

4. Begin by telling members to relax and let their thoughts flow freely in and out of their minds as they concentrate on your voice.
5. Ask them to focus their breathing as it is happening naturally. Become aware of their inhalations and exhalations, of the rising and falling of their chests (allow 2–3 minutes).
6. Ask them to relax each body part, one at a time (allow 2–3 minutes).
7. Ask them to expel any remaining stress left in their body with each exhalation (allow 2–3 minutes).
8. Members should now be relaxed. Proceed with the following exercises (resume regular breathing in between each):
    a. Deep breathing from the diaphragm.
    b. Full inhalation with breath holding for as long as possible.
    c. Bone breathing—breathing into different parts of the body.
    d. Breathing as slowly as possible.
    e. Breathing in through the nose and out through the mouth.
    f. Exhaling any unwanted thoughts or feelings until they are all gone.
    g. In sitting position at a table members practice breathing with a steady air stream by blowing a candle flame and trying to keep it at a 45-degree angle.

F. Tension-relaxation exercises.
1. While seated, members get into a relaxed position with their eyes closed and tense and release each body part as you call them out one by one—go through the entire body.
2. Explain how tensing and relaxing body parts helps the body to relax through biofeedback and body awareness.

G. Process the exercises.
1. Members identify and discuss the exercise that was most effective in their relaxation.
2. Members discuss positive experiences and how they felt before and after the exercises.
3. Members discuss uncomfortable experiences and how they felt before and after the exercises.

H. Members state where and when they could perform these techniques at home.

I. Members state how these exercises could be helpful in preventing a relapse and/or gaining sobriety.

J. *Homework*:
Members will practice these relaxation techniques daily and report their progress in next session.

STRESS MANAGEMENT

Day ____________________

Group Leader Plan

Anger Management

I. *Objectives*: Members will be able to:
   A. Define "anger management."
   B. Discuss and understand the negative effects if anger is not managed properly.
   C. Discuss how drugs and alcohol affect anger.
   D. List healthy ways of dealing with their angry feelings.
   E. List unhealthy ways of dealing with their angry feelings.
   F. Monitor when they are angry through identifying their signs and symptoms of anger.
   G. Identify things that make them angry.
   H. Identify new anger management skills that they would like to practice.
   I. Keep an anger management journal and report on their progress.

II. *Materials*: Form 3-8, Form 3-9, Form 3-10, blackboard, chalk, and pens.

III. *Procedures*:
   A. Form 3-8, "Anger Management."
      1. Distribute.
      2. Have members read it aloud, discussing it as they go.
   B. Form 3-9, "Anger Management Worksheet."
      1. Distribute.
      2. Have members read it aloud.
      3. Any questions?
      4. Allow time for completion.
      5. Discuss their answers.
      6. List their answers on the board under "healthy" or "unhealthy" ways to deal with anger.
   C. *Homework*:
      Form 3-10, "Anger Management Journal."
      1. Distribute.
      2. Have members read it aloud.
      3. Any questions?
      4. Discuss similarity to Form 3-6, "Stress Management Journal," completed in a prior session.
      5. Members are to complete as much as possible at home until next session, when they will discuss their progress.
      6. Instruct members to use their responses to #5 on their Form 3-9, "Anger Management Worksheet," in the space provided for new ways to deal with anger.

Anger Management

Anger is a natural feeling that all humans experience. It does not have to be a negative feeling. However, it can get us into a lot of trouble if it is not dealt with in a healthy way.

"*Anger management*" means dealing with angry feelings in a positive way. One of the first steps in learning how to do this is to be able to know what makes you angry. It also helps to know when you are angry. Many people with substance abuse problems do not know when they are angry because for years drugs/alcohol have covered up their angry feelings. Once clean, they may not be aware of their anger or what causes it. But, the anger is still there underneath everything. When anger is stored up this way, several negative things can happen:

1. People can become angry over little things.
2. They can develop explosive outbursts.
3. They can turn their anger inward, resulting in depression or withdrawal.
4. They can "act out" by doing destructive acts against themselves.
5. They can take their anger out on someone else.
6. Anger can be a trigger because some people use substances to manage their anger.

People with mental health problems also may have difficulty expressing their angry feelings.

1. They may not be assertive enough due to low self-confidence.
2. They may end up doing what other people want and swallow their own anger.
3. They may be very sensitive to rejection.
4. They may fear rejection if they express negative feelings.

Many of these things go on without people being aware of them. So, you can see why it is important to develop new ways to effectively deal with your anger. We talk about anger management in the stress management topic, because if you can cope with your angry feelings, you may feel less stress in your daily lives.

ANGER MANAGEMENT HELPS DECREASE STRESS
MANAGING YOUR ANGER KEEPS YOU FROM USING DRUGS/ALCOHOL

Form 3-9

Anger Management Worksheet

1. List below:

Healthy Ways to Deal with Anger	*Unhealthy Ways to Deal with Anger*

2. I know I am angry when ______________________________
____
______________________________.

(These are my signs and symptoms of anger).

3. The following things really make me angry ______________________________
____
______________________________.

4. When I get angry, I ______________________________
____
______________________________.

(These are ways with which I deal with anger now).

5. I would like to learn or practice the following anger management skills ________
____
____
______________________________.

6. *Homework*: I will keep an anger management journal until next session. I will discuss my progress with anger management in the next session.

Form 3-10

Anger Management Journal

	Event That Made Me Angry	*What I Did*	*New Anger Management Techniques I Could Try*
Monday			
Tuesday			
Wednesday			
Thursday			
Friday			
Saturday			
Sunday			

STRESS MANAGEMENT

Day ________________

Group Leader Plan

Stretching Exercises

I. *Objectives*: Members will be able to:
   A. Locate muscular tension in their bodies.
   B. Stretch different parts of their bodies.
   C. State how daily stretching can relieve tension.
   D. Identify a time and place to practice daily stretching and set a goal to do so on their own.
   E. Report progress in using this stress management technique.

II. *Materials*: Form 3-11; Form 3-12; mats; large, quiet room with floor space, energizing music, tables or chairs for balance; loose, comfortable clothes.

III. *Procedures*:
   A. Teach how daily stretching relieves muscular tension.
      1. Form 3-11, "The Twelve Steps of Stretching."
         a. Distribute.
         b. Have members read it aloud.
         c. Lead a short discussion about the physiology of the muscles, tendons, and storage of tension. Explain how stretching decreases muscle bulk and releases calcium and magnesium to the blood stream, which promotes relaxation.
   B. Injury prevention.
      1. Form 3-12, "Stretching—Injury Prevention."
         a. Have members read aloud.
         b. Ask if anyone who has a current injury or heart problem feels they should not participate.
   C. Demonstrate stretching exercises.
      1. Ask if any members can demonstrate a stretch and tell what muscles he or she has affected. Have everyone do it together.
      2. Demonstrate any stretches that they did not mention. Have the group do them. Try to have people hold each of them for 30 seconds. After each stretch ask members to point out the muscles affected. Ask how people feel after each.
         a. Neck rolls (sitting).
            - Drop head forward.
            - Drop head back.
            - Touch left ear to left shoulder.
            - Touch right ear to right shoulder.
            - Roll whole head clockwise slowly.
            - Roll whole head counterclockwise slowly.

b. Face relaxation (sitting).
    - Allow face muscles to relax so that the jaw drops.
    - Protrude tongue outward as far as possible.
    - Roll eyes from left to right.
    - Roll eyes up then down.
    - Roll eyes in a clockwise direction.
    - Roll eyes in a counterclockwise direction.

c. Calf stretches (standing against a wall).
    - Lean into the wall with arms bent but legs straight.
    - Feel the tension on the back of the legs.
    - Hold and release.

d. Quadriceps stretches (standing near a chair or table for support).
    - Bend the knee of one leg.
    - Grab foot with same side hand.
    - Stretch leg up so foot reaches your hip.

e. Side stretches (standing).
    - Raise one arm above your head.
    - Stretch your body over to the right side.
    - Stretch your body over to the left side.

f. Toe touches (standing).
    - Bend body forward at the waist with knees straight.
    - Go down as far as possible.
    - Bend knees.
    - Go down farther.
    - Straighten knees.

D. *Homework*:
Members will verbalize a goal to practice stretching between now and next session. They will report their progress in the next session.

Form 3-11

The Twelve Steps of Stretching

1. We admitted that we have stress in our lives.

2. We came to believe that stretching exercises would help relieve our daily tension.

3. We made a decision to stretch daily.

4. We have taken inventory of our bodies to identify stress where we store tension.

5. We admitted these areas to our group members.

6. We were entirely ready to have stretching exercises remove all of our bodily tension.

7. We humbly asked for a demonstration on how to stretch properly.

8. We made a list of all the people we had harmed due to our own stress, and became willing to manage our stress in healthier ways.

9. We made amends to such people wherever possible, and share with them our new goal.

10. We continued to monitor our bodies for signs of muscular tension. When we allowed our tension to build up we admitted it.

11. We sought, through stretching exercises, to improve our daily lives.

12. Having gained a new stress management technique as a result of these steps, we tried to teach this technique to other dual diagnosis members, and practice them ourselves in our daily lives.

Modified from: *Alcoholics Anonymous*, 3rd ed. New York: AA World Services, 59–60.

Stretching—Injury Prevention

1. Stretch slowly.

2. Do not bounce.

3. Do not force a movement that will not go.

4. Stop if you feel sharp pain.

5. Do not overexert yourself.

6. Do not execute exercises if you have a serious heart condition or a current injury.

7. Try not to eat any food before stretching. Food makes it harder to stretch because your body is digesting it.

8. Have fun.

STRESS MANAGEMENT

Day ____________________

Group Leader Plan

Dealing with Difficult Family Situations

I. *Objectives*: Members will be able to:
   A. Identify a stressful family situation.
   B. Describe their behavior in this situation.
   C. Problem solve through role playing.
   D. Increase ability to deal with stressful family situations by practicing solutions at home.

II. *Materials*: Form 3-13 and pens.

III. *Procedures*:
   A. Form 3-13, "Dealing with Difficult Family Situations."
      1. Distribute.
      2. Have members read it aloud.
      3. Ask them to complete questions 1 and 2.
      4. Any questions?
      5. Allow time for completion.
   B. Role play to problem solve stressful situations.
      1. One member at a time describes their difficult family situation in question 1 on their handout.
      2. The member then describes how they usually deal with it, and why this works or doesn't work.
      3. The member assigns volunteers to role play the situation using a different way to deal with the stress.
      4. Discuss the role play and what was learned from it. Have the member record what they have learned in question 4.
      5. Repeat the whole role play sequence 1–4 with every member.
   C. *Homework*:
      Each member will use the new stress management ideas they listed in number 4 to better manage difficult family situations at home.

Dealing with Difficult Family Situations

1. Describe a family interaction which causes you stress.

2. Describe how you usually deal with it.

3. Ask members from the group to role play your situation to problem solve different ways of dealing with the stress.

4. Given what you learned from the role play, what would you do differently next time this situation arises?

STRESS MANAGEMENT

Day ________________

Group Leader Plan

Biofeedback

I. *Objectives*: Members will be able to:
   A. Define "biofeedback."
   B. Give three examples of biofeedback techniques to reduce stress.
   C. Discuss how these techniques can reduce stress.
   D. Monitor their heart rate.
   E. Monitor their breath rate.
   F. Monitor their body tension.
   G. Use biofeedback independently as a stress management technique.

II. *Materials*: Form 3-14, mirrors, a quiet room, stethoscope (optional), and pens.

III. *Procedures*:
   A. Form 3-14, "Biofeedback."
      1. Distribute.
      2. Have members read it aloud.
      3. Any comments or questions?
   B. Heart rate.
      1. Demonstrate how to take a heart rate at rest (sitting still).
      2. Have members take and record their own resting heart rate.
      3. Lead the group in a short exercise to raise their heart rates.
      4. Have members take and record their heart rates immediately following the exercise.
      5. Conduct a group relaxation technique where members keep a finger on their pulse and try to decrease their heart rate to as low as possible.
      6. Members now take and record their heart rates after trying to lower it.
      7. Members can work with partners monitoring their partner's heart rate if time allows.
   C. Breath rate.
      1. Repeat steps 1–7 under heart rate above, but this time measure and record breath rate (how many breaths taken per minute).
   D. Facial tension.
      1. Have members look at themselves in a mirror.
      2. Have them observe their facial features, noting and

recording if they are relaxed or tense.

3. Have members try to relax the facial features that appear tense. Ask them to feel the difference.
4. Members can work in pairs if time allows instead of using the mirrors. One member gives feedback about the other's facial tension while the other tries to relax that particular part. Members watching indicate whether their partners succeeded in relaxing their faces.

E. *Homework*:
Members will practice using biofeedback techniques to better manage their stress. They will report their progress next session.

Form 3-14

Biofeedback

Bio refers to body and *feedback* means to receive information about yourself. So, *biofeedback* means to receive information about yourself from your body. Your body can tell you what is going on with it if you know how to listen.

We are going to ask our bodies about our level of stress. We will learn how to listen for the answers. Our bodies can constantly tell about our level of stress. We can decide at any time to tune in and listen, then use this information to regulate our bodies so we feel more relaxed. Sound complicated? Maybe, because people who abuse substances become unaware of their bodies:

1. They feel numb or detached.
2. They are unable to listen to signals.

Drugs and alcohol also change the body's signals so the wrong message gets sent.

Luckily for us, it is easy to relearn to read the body's signals. Let's look at a few examples:

1. Heart Rate.
   At rest ________________
   After exercise ________________
   After relaxation technique ________________

2. Breath Rate.
   At rest ________________
   After exercise ________________
   After relaxation technique ________________

3. Facial Tension.
   Check below

	Relaxed?	or	Tense?
Eye brows			
Forehead			
Lips			
Jaw			
Eyes			

STRESS MANAGEMENT

Day____________________

Group Leader Plan

Nutrition

I. *Objectives*: Members will be able to:
   A. State how proper nutrition can help manage stress.
   B. List foods and liquids that can increase anxiety.
   C. Explain why these foods and liquids can increase anxiety.
   D. Identify problems with their nutritional habits.
   E. Set a goal to better manage stress by improving one poor eating habit.

II. *Materials*: Form 3-15, Form 3-16, and pens.

III. *Procedures*:
   A. Form 3-15, "Nutrition."
      1. Distribute.
      2. Have members read it aloud.
      3. Pause after each number for questions, clarification, problems, or specific life examples.
   B. Form 3-16, "Foods or Liquids That Can Make You Anxious."
      1. Distribute.
      2. Have members read it aloud.
      3. Any questions?
      4. Allow time for completion.
      5. Discuss their answers.
         Stimulants.
            Examples of stimulants:
               Coffee
               Tea
               Soda
               Red pepper spice
            Effects of stimulants:
               Stimulants like caffeine or natural stimulants cause the body to speed up its functions and can result in feeling anxious.
            Examples of foods containing chemicals:
               Butter on the popcorn from theater
               Hot dogs
            Effects of chemicals:
               Chemical additives in food can cause allergies and hyperactivity.
               Some are poisons. Red dye #2 was found to cause cancer.
               Monosodium glutamate (MSG) may cause headaches.

Salt.

Examples of foods high in salt:

Sardines
Olives
Ham
Chinese food
Anchovies
Canned vegetables
Canned soups

Effects of a diet high in salt:

Salt causes fluid retention in the body. The cells can no longer eliminate wastes and absorb nutrients as fast as normally required.

The body feels bloated. You become irritable and anxious.

Sugar.

Examples of foods high in sugar:

Candy
Donuts
Pie
Cake
A lot of fruits or fruit juices

Effects of a diet high in sugar:

Sugars increase anxiety if they are fast metabolizing sugars such as all the ones listed. They cause a surge of energy and a rise in insulin. After 15 minutes or so, they cause a sharp decline in energy level and insulin. This leaves the body depleted. Many people fall asleep after eating a lot of sugar.

C. Have members identify problems with their current nutritional habits.

D. From their problem, have members each set a goal to improve their nutrition to better manage their stress.

E. *Homework*:
Members will follow through with their goals above and report on their progress in the next session.

Nutrition

How Good Nutrition Helps Manage Stress

1. Anxiety burns calories. If the extra calories are not added back throughout the day, the body starts burning stored energy. The body becomes depleted of energy and the following starts to happen:
    a. Light headedness.
    b. Dizziness.
    c. Difficulty concentrating.
    d. Increased anxiety.
    e. Fatigue.
    f. Irritability.
    g. Poor decision making ability.
    h. Poor problem solving.

2. Anxiety produces more acid in the stomach. If there is no food in the stomach, the extra acid can begin to wear away the lining of the stomach walls. Over time an ulcer can occur.

3. Allowing yourself time to eat breakfast, lunch, and dinner daily builds in relaxation. It breaks up your day. It give you something to look forward to. It offers a break from work or your programs.

4. Eating can be social. Talking or sharing time with people can decrease stress.

5. Your body needs appropriate nutrients to handle daily stress whether it be physical or mental. You have heard of "stress reducing" vitamins. The "B" vitamins have been shown to help the body deal with stress if taken regularly.

6. Stress lowers your immune system. When your immune system is low, your body becomes susceptible to illness. You begin to feel run down and may actually become ill. Three balanced meals are required each day to keep your immune system strong during times of stress.

7. An empty stomach can cause drug/alcohol cravings, so keep your belly full!

Form 3-16

Foods or Liquids That Can Make You Anxious

Do you know why?

Coffee

Tea

Soda

Candy

Donuts

Popcorn from the theater

Pie

Cake

Red pepper spice

Hot dogs

A lot of fruit or fruit juice

Sardines

Olives

Chinese food

Ham

Pickles

Canned soup

Anchovies

Canned vegetables

Avoiding these will help manage stress. Managing stress helps you stay sober.

STRESS MANAGEMENT

Day___________________

Group Leader Plan

Poetry, Music, and Crafts

I. *Objectives*: Members will be able to:
   A. State how poetry, music, and crafts can manage stress.
   B. Use poetry, music, and crafts as stress management techniques.
   C. Make a reference list of music and crafts that help relax them and refer to it when needed.

II. *Materials*: Form 3-17, Form 3-18, poetry, relaxing music, paper, and pens.

III. *Procedures*:
   A. Poetry relaxation exercise.
      1. Have members sit around table with paper and pens.
      2. Create a relaxing atmosphere with music in the background.
      3. Explain that you are going to read poetry and ask members to concentrate on the words of the poem and try to relax.
      4. Read several relaxing poems.
      5. Ask members to write something of their own. You can identify a theme.
      6. Have members share their writings.
      7. Have members discuss the experience.
   B. Form 3-17, "Activities and Relaxation."
      1. Distribute.
      2. Have members read it aloud.
      3. Any questions?
      4. Allow time for completion.
      5. Instruct members to transfer their "relaxing" activities from this handout to #1 in the second handout entitled "Personal Stress Reducers."
   C. Form 3-18, "Personal Stress Reducers."
      1. Distribute.
      2 Have members read it aloud.
      3. Any questions?
      4. Allow time for completion.
      5. Discuss their answers.
      6. Emphasize that this is a reference sheet for members to refer to when they feel stressed.

D. *Homework*:
Members will refer to today's handout, "Personal Stress Reducers," when they feel stress between now and next session. They are to choose one of the stress management techniques that they recorded today and use it to better manage their stresses.

Activities and Relaxation

Please rate each activity according to how relaxing, neutral, or stressful it is for you.

Activity	Relaxing	Neutral	Stressful
Reading			
Walking			
Socializing			
Playing cards			
Swimming			
Singing			
Drawing			
Making craft projects			
Painting			
Woodworking			
Dancing			
Exercising			
Sewing			
Talking on the telephone			
Watching TV			
Going to a movie			
Museums			
Libraries			
Listening to music			
Computer games			
Others (list below)			

Form 3-18

Personal Stress Reducers

Refer to this sheet when you feel stress.

1. List below activities, crafts, or hobbies that can help decrease your stress.

    a.

    b.

    c.

    d.

    e.

    f.

2. List below specific songs, music, types of music, or radio stations that help you relax.

    a.

    b.

    c.

    d.

    e.

    f.

3. What smells are relaxing to you?

    a.

    b.

    c.

    d.

STRESS MANAGEMENT

Day____________________

Group Leader Plan

Summary of My Stress Reducers

I. *Objective*: Members will be able to:
   A. Review their workbook materials.
   B. List the stress management techniques that have worked the most effectively for them throughout the course.
   C. Utilize this summary reference sheet of personal stress management techniques as needed in their daily lives.

II. *Materials*: Form 3-19 and pens.

III. *Procedures*:
   A. Form 3-19, "Summary of My Stress Reducers."
      1. Distribute.
      2. Have members read it aloud.
      3. Any questions?
      4. Allow time for completion.
      5. Review their answers.
   B. *Homework*:
      Members will refer to this sheet when they feel stressed or want to use drugs or alcohol. They will choose an appropriate stress management technique, use it, and report their progress next session.

Form 3-19

Summary of My Stress Reducers

Go through your Living Skills Recovery workbook to review all the stress management techniques you have learned so far. List below all the ones that helped you throughout this topic. This is your summary reference sheet. When you feel stressed or get cravings you should always refer back to this sheet and choose an appropriate technique.

Manage Your Stress!   Stay Clean and Sober!

1.

2.

3.

4.

5.

6.

7.

8.

9.

10.

11.

12.

13.

14.

4 Social Skills for Sobriety

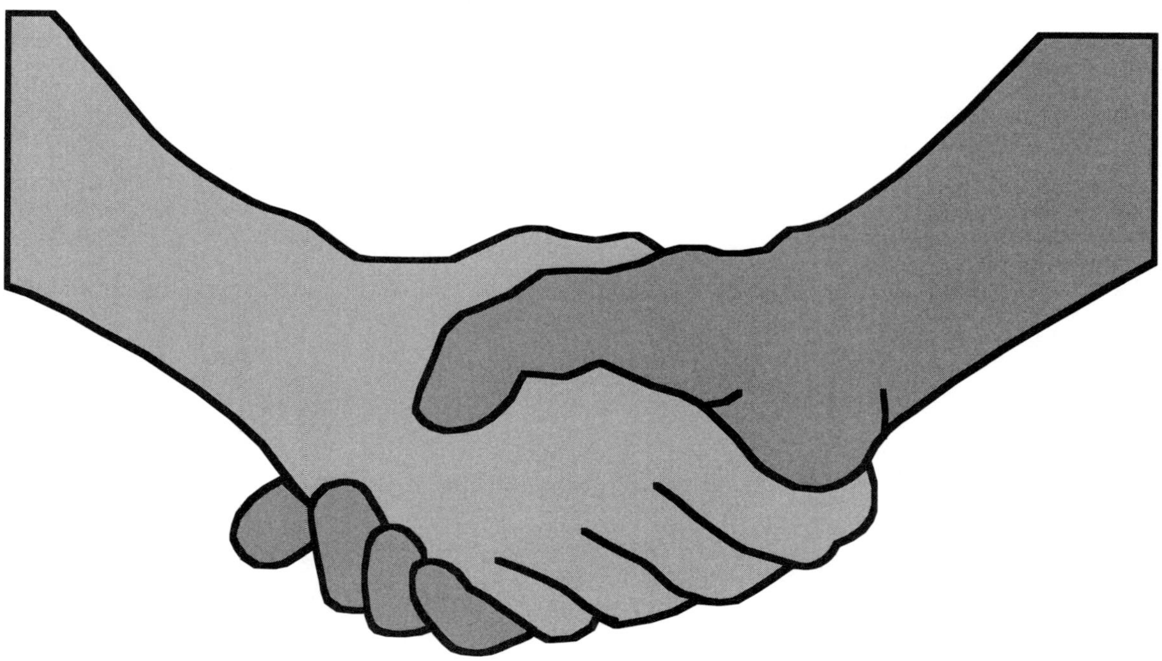

SOCIAL SKILLS

Day ___________________

Group Leader Plan

Social Skills: Strengths and Problem Areas

I. *Objectives*: Members will be able to:
   A. Identify some of their strengths in social skills.
   B. Identify some of their deficits in social skills.
   C. Identify which of these deficits they would like to improve during this group.
   D. Increase their understanding of why it is important for them to strengthen their social skills given their dual diagnoses.

II. *Materials*: Form 4-1 and pens.

II. *Procedures*:
   A. Form 4-1, "Social Skills Strengths and Problem Areas."
      1. Distribute.
      2. Have members read it aloud.
      3. Any questions?
      4. Allow time for completion.
      5. Discuss their answers.

Social Skills Strengths and Problem Areas

We will be spending the next group of sessions practicing and discussing social skills.

Everyone needs social contacts. Often people in recovery from drug addiction need to make new friends and acquaintances who do not use drugs. It is easier to maintain sobriety this way. You may have clean time, but having additional social supports on the outside will help you make a smoother transition to your community when you are ready to move on.

There are many social skills that can help you maintain sobriety:

1. Being able to say "no."
2. Being assertive.
3. Anger management.
4. Being able to receive feedback.
5. Being aware of your feelings.

How can these skills help?

When people have a mental illness, they often have problems with the following social skills:

1. Feeling good about themselves.
2. Being assertive.
3. Decision making.
4. Meeting new people.
5. Adjusting to change.

Why do you think these might be difficult?

Keeping in mind all the social skills we have mentioned today:

1. Which ones are you good at?

2. Which ones are you are *not* good at?

3. Which ones would you like to work on in this group?

SOCIAL SKILLS

Day____________________

Group Leader Plan

A Picture Is Worth a Thousand Words*

I. *Objectives*: Members will be able to:
   A. Define and give examples of observation skills.
   B. Recognize how observation skills are important to social skills.
   C. Develop an awareness of their own body language.
   D. Develop an awareness of other people's body language.

II. *Materials*: Forms 4-2 and 4-3 cut into individual cards, Group Leader Plan, "Observation Skill Cards Answers," jar or container for cards, and one index card marked "wink."

III. *Procedures*:
   A. Therapeutic exercise "wink."
      1. Acquisition—everyone sits in a circle so members can all see each other. Members pick folded pieces of paper from a jar. All of the pieces of paper are blank except one, which is marked "wink." Members should not show each other their cards. The member with the "wink" card is to begin winking at other members one by one, discretely but making direct eye contact each time. Within 30 seconds after a member has been winked at, they are to close their eyes and lower their head until the game is over. Everyone who has not been winked at should try to guess who the winker is. Each member has two guesses.
      2. Purpose:
         - to discover how people use their eyes to communicate.
         - to increase eye contact.
   B. Therapeutic exercise "shopping."
      1. Acquisition—Members all sit in a circle so everyone can see each other. Group leader says, "I am going to use the phrase 'I went shopping and bought . . .'" and you are to fill it in with something you make up. I will tell you if "you did" or if "you did not." The group members take turns with answering the same phrase. During the game, the members try to figure out the rule behind the leader's decision of "yes you did" or "no you did not." It is based on whether or not the person answering the question has their legs crossed or not. You may use variations of similar body presentations such as crossed arms, but it must be something everyone can see.

2. Purpose:
    - to demonstrate the areas of the body that are used to communicate attitudes and moods.
    - to increase awareness of body language.

C. Therapeutic exercise "feelings."
1. Acquisition—Write the name of a feeling on a card. Have as many different cards as members. Each member randomly selects a card. Without showing their cards to others, the members take turns acting out the feeling using only non-verbal gestures and facial expressions, while others guess what it is. The winner goes next to demonstrate the feeling on his or her card.
2. Purpose—subtle observation skills:
    a. Identify different body parts which portray different feelings.
    b. Identify how these body parts change in relation to different feelings.
    c. Be able to communicate a feeling to others without speaking.
    d. Increase overall awareness of subtle observation skills.
    e. Practice different facial expressions.

D. Vignettes—Form 4-2, "Observation Skill Cards."
1. Acquisition—Pass out one card at a time to a member. Have that member read his or her card aloud and try to answer it with help from the group. You may check the members' answers with the answers given in the Group Leader Plan, "Observation Skill Cards Answers."
2. Purpose—Increase problem solving by applying newly learned observation skills to familiar, real life situations.

E. *Homework*:
Form 4-3, "Observation Skill Homework Cards."
1. Acquisition—Pass out one card at a time to each member. Each member takes turns reading a card aloud and trying to answer it. If they cannot answer it correctly, they have it for homework.
2. Purpose—Increase observation skills in members' home environment and neighborhood.

*Modified from Bond, T. *Games for Social and Life Skills.* London: Hutchinson and Co., 1986, pp. 147–148.

SOCIAL SKILLS

Day__________________

Group Leader Plan

Observation Skill Cards Answers

You have something to say in a 12-step meeting, but there are a lot of people attending. How do you get called on?

- Sit where people can see you.
- Raise your hand very high while sitting up straight during a quiet time.
- Keep trying.
- Raise your hand quickly and strongly.

How do you let someone know you have heard what they said in a conversation?

1. Nod your head.
2. Make eye contact.
3. Say an occasional "yes."
4. Paraphrase when they finish.
5. Continue the topic of conversation.

How can you tell if someone is friendly or not?

Open Posture (friendly)	versus	Closed Posture (unfriendly)
• Eye contact.		• No eye contact.
• Smiling.		• Frown.
• Forward lean.		• Head down.
• Arms open or gesturing.		• Crossed arms and/or legs.
		• Person looks away when you make eye contact.

How do you speak so that people will want to listen to you?

- Loud enough.
- In a crisp voice.
- Direct your voice to different people in the room.
- Use eye contact.
- Chin up, head up.
- Use facial expressions or gestures for emphasis.

How can you tell when someone is on drugs?

- Red eyes.
- Change in behavior:
  - quiet/withdrawn or hyperactive
  - anxious
  - asleep more often.
- Change pupils.
- Inappropriate behavior.
- If you don't see them in their groups.

How do you know if someone is listening to you during a conversation?

If they:

1. Make eye contact.
2. Use head nods.
3. Can paraphrase when you finish.
4. Ask appropriate questions.
5. Continue the topic of conversation.
6. Say occasional "yes."

You are refusing drugs from someone. How do you show you mean "*NO*" when you say "*NO*"?

1. Say "no" and walk away quickly, abruptly.
2. Say "no" in a strong voice without hesitation.
3. Do not make eye contact.
4. Ignore them if they ask again or try to pursue you.
5. Use hand gestures moving away from your body.

Form 4-2

Observation Skill Cards

You have something to say in your 12-step meeting, but there are a lot of people attending. How do you get called on?	How do you let someone know you have heard what they said in a conversation?
How can you tell who is friendly and who is not?	How do you speak so that people will want to listen to you?
How can you tell when someone is on drugs?	How do you know if someone is listening to you during a conversation?
You are refusing drugs from someone. How do you show you mean "*NO*" when you say "*NO*"?	

Observation Skill Homework Cards

What colors are the doors to your program?	What office number is your therapist in?
What is the name of the nearest grocery store in your neighborhood?	What color is your bathroom?
What is your therapist wearing today?	What colors are the second hands on the clocks?
Where is the nearest bus stop to your apartment? Where does that bus go?	What was the weather like this morning?

SOCIAL SKILLS

Day____________________

Group Leader Plan

Starting a Conversation

I. *Objectives*: Members will be able to:
   A. Generate ten appropriate conversation starters.
   B. State the difference between open-ended and closed-ended questions, and be able to write examples of each.
   C. Practice using these new conversation starters with other members, family, friends, and people whom they have never met before in their community.
   D. State how meeting new people is important to their recovery.

II. *Materials*: Form 4-4 and pens.

II. Procedures:
   A. Form 4-4, "Conversation Starters."
      1. Distribute.
      2. Have members read it aloud.
      3. Any questions?
      4. Allow time for completion.
      5. Discuss their answers.
   B. Define open-ended and close-ended questions.
      1. Open-ended—A question which can *never* be answered by just one word.[1]
      2. Closed-ended—A question which *can* be answered by just one word.[1]
   C. Have members reread their conversation starters and state whether they are "open-" or "closed-ended questions."
   D. Have members rewrite all of their closed-ended questions and make them open-ended.
   E. Have members role play two people having a conversation beginning with one of their open-ended conversation starters. See if it generates more than a few sentences.
   F. Which conversation starters could you say to someone you have never met before?
   G. Homework.
      Practice starting conversations using your new "conversation starters" with:
      1. Another member.
      2. A family member.
      3. A friend/acquaintance outside the program.
      4. Someone you have never spoken to before in your community.

H. Discuss why meeting new people is important in recovery.
   1. You need to meet new drug free people in order to stay away from people, places, and things.
   2. Loneliness can be a trigger.
   3. Meeting people in your group increases your participation.
   4. You can get support and learn from others.

Form 4-4

Conversation Starters

List ten different sentences you could say to begin a conversation.

1.

2.

3.

4.

5.

6.

7.

8.

9.

10.

*Modified with permission from Schwimmer-Stern, P. Life Skills Curriculum (unpublished master's project), 1986.

SOCIAL SKILLS

Day__________________

Group Leader Plan

The Gift of Gab

I. *Objectives*: Members will be able to:
   A. Keep a conversation going.
   B. Converse in a group one-to-one.
   C. Judge who is appropriate and who is inappropriate for extended conversation.
   D. Distinguish inappropriate topics (those which are too personal) from appropriate topics of conversation.
   E. Identify what makes it difficult for them to keep a conversation going and problem solve around their difficulties.
   F. Increase communication with service providers.

II. *Materials*: Blackboard and chalk.

III. *Procedures*:
   A. Therapeutic game "Finding Your Voice."
      1. Demonstrate with one other group member, then have members work in dyad.
      2. Both people begin speaking at the same time about anything, it does not have to make sense. Both people keep talking nonstop without a break and without listening to each other. The game ends when one member stops talking. The other is the winner.
      3. Purpose:
         a. Getting used to the feeling of talking a lot in a nonthreatening game.
         b. To serve as an icebreaker to more difficult exercises.
   B. List on the board as members call out what types of people are appropriate for an extended conversation and who are not and why.
   C. List on the board as members call out what topics are good for extended conversations and which are not. Examples include:

Personal Topics	versus	General, Factual Topics
family problems		movies
details about your physical health		TV shows
your treatment		music
		current events

   D. Redefine and remind members to:
      1. Use open-ended questions to generate material for discussion.
      2. Listen and take turns talking.

3. Remember to observe body language and social cues during the conversation in order to keep the conversation active.

E. Role play—generating conversation.
   1. In dyads without the group leader.
      a. Divide members into dyads.
      b. Have each dyad choose a topic.
      c. Have all dyads engage in a conversation at the same time.
   2. In front of the group with the group leader and two other members demonstrate a three-way conversation around a given topic.
   3. In front of the group with the group leader and one other member repeat step 2, but with two people.
   4. In front of the group with two members (no group leader). The purpose of the sequence above is to grade the activity from simple to more difficult.

F. List on the board as members call out what makes it difficult for them to keep a conversation going, for example, shy, self-conscious, poor conversation skills, difficult listening, impatience.

G. Problem solve how to get over these obstacles, for example, practice or converse around an activity of common interest.

H. Discussing humor in conversation. How does it help?
   1. Relieves tension so that the conversation can continue.
   2. Breaks the ice.
   3. Helps people relate on a similar, universal level.
   4. Breaks through stereotypes and cultures.
   5. Helps people feel closer to each other.
   6. Makes people happy.

SOCIAL SKILLS

Day__________________

Group Leader Plan

Finishing a Conversation

I. *Objectives*: Members will be able to:
   A. Finish a conversation.
   B. Make further arrangements to meet with that person at another time.
   C. State the benefits of completing a conversation and making new plans.

II. *Materials*: None.

III. *Procedures*: Members will role play ending a conversation they have started.
   A. Role playing.
      1. Members will begin a conversation using open-ended questions.
      2. Members will keep the conversations going using paraphrasing, body language, active listening, and requests for clarification.
      3. Members will practice ending the conversation with further plans to get together in the future.

SOCIAL SKILLS

Day ________________

Group Leader Plan

Where to Meet New People

I. *Objectives*: Members will be able to:
   A. Review where they have met people in the past.
   B. Identify new places they could go to meet people who are drug and alcohol free.
   C. Practice meeting new people on the outside using the techniques discussed in this and in previous sessions.

II. *Materials*: Form 4-5 and pens.

III. *Procedures*:
   A. Form 4-5, "Meeting New People."
      1. Distribute.
      2. Have members read it aloud.
      3. Any questions?
      4. Allow time for completion.
      5. Discuss their answers.

Meeting New People

1. What are some places people in general go to meet new people?

2. Where did you meet your best friend?

3. Where have you met people in the past?

4. What *new* places could *you* go to in the future to meet new people who are drug/alcohol free?

5. Choose one new place you listed in #4. List it below. Between now and next session, go there and practice meeting new people using the techniques we have talked about in previous sessions.

SOCIAL SKILLS

Day ____________________

Group Leader Plan

Self-Esteem*

I. *Objectives*: Members will be able to:
   A. List positive attributes characteristic of themselves and of other group members.
   B. Learn new positive attributes about themselves that other people see in them, but that they are not aware of.
   C. Begin to rebuild their self-esteem which drugs or alcohol have stripped away, and which has been damaged by the stigma of having a mental illness.
   D. Be able to accept compliments.
   E. Be able to compliment others.
   F. Get to know themselves better.

II. *Materials*: Form 4-6 and pens.

III. *Procedures*:
   A. Form 4-6, "Self-Esteem."
      1. Distribute.
      2. Have members read it aloud.
      3. Explain purpose of handout (see objectives above).
      4. Ask members to fill in the blanks with a positive attribute about themselves which begins with the letter indicated.
      5. Any questions?
      6. Allow time for completion.
      7. Discuss their answers. If members cannot think of some attributes, other members may help them out.

*Modified with permission from Korb, K. L., Azok, S., and Leutenberg, E. A. *Life Management Skills I.* Beachwood, OH: Wellness Reproductions, Inc., 1993, p. 35.

Self-Esteem

Hey, hey, say I'm pretty cool.
Say, I'm no fool.
I wanna be strong.
And I wanna live long.
Ain't nobody mess with me,
Cuz I like myself A through Z!

A. ______________________________
B. ______________________________
C. ______________________________
D. ______________________________
E. ______________________________
F. ______________________________
G. ______________________________
H. ______________________________
I. ______________________________
J. ______________________________
K. ______________________________
L. ______________________________
M. ______________________________
N. ______________________________
O. ______________________________
P. ______________________________
Q. ______________________________
R. ______________________________
S. ______________________________
T. ______________________________
U. ______________________________
V. ______________________________
W. ______________________________
X. ______________________________
Y. ______________________________
Z. ______________________________

*Modified with permission from Korb, K. L., Azok, S., and Leutenberg, E. A. *Life Management Skills I.* Beachwood, OH: Wellness Reproductions, Inc., 1993, p. 35.

SOCIAL SKILLS

Day________________

Group Leader Plan

Self-Awareness

I. *Objectives*: Members will be able to:
   A. Begin to take a moral inventory (step 4 of the 12-step program) of their lives.
   B. Become more aware of their attitudes, values, feelings, strengths, and weaknesses.
   C. Share A and B with the group.

II. *Materials*: Form 4-7 and pens.

III. *Procedures*:
   A. Form 4-7, "Self-Awareness."
      1. Ask members if any of them have begun working on the fourth step yet.
      2. Explain the purpose of the exercise and introduce step 4.
      3. Distribute.
      4. Allow time for completion.
      5. Discuss their answers.

Self Awareness

1. Because of drinking/drugging I ______________________________.
2. The thing I dislike most about myself is ______________________________.
3. When I got high/drunk I used to ______________________________.
4. My worst fear now is ______________________________.
5. I used to be afraid when ______________________________.
6. I get really angry when ______________________________.
7. I am the type of person that ______________________________.
8. My higher power ______________________________.
9. I like myself when/because ______________________________.
10. It is hard for me to say "no" when ______________________________.
11. When someone tells me what to do I ______________________________.
12. I feel rejected when ______________________________.
13. When someone puts me down I ______________________________.
14. I can hardly wait until ______________________________.
15. If I had my way, I would ______________________________.
16. I miss ______________________________.
17. If I were ten years old, I would ______________________________.
18. It takes a lot of courage to ______________________________.
19. I would like to ______________________________.

SOCIAL SKILLS

Day ________________

Group Leader Plan

Assertiveness Training*

I. *Objectives*: Members will be able to:
   A. Define "passive," "assertive," and "aggressive" behavior.
   B. Distinguish between the three.
   C. Identify their own behaviors as either passive, assertive, or aggressive.
   D. Role play a given situation each of the three different ways (passively, assertively, and aggressively) in order to begin to change their pattern of response.
   E. State one way acting assertively can aid in their recovery, in managing stress, and in improving social skills.
   F. State and follow through with a goal to be more assertive.

II. *Materials*: Form 4-8 and pens.

III. *Procedures*:
   A. Form 4-8, "Assertiveness Training."
      1. Distribute.
      2. Have members read it aloud.
      3. Any questions?
      4. Allow time for completion.
      5. Discuss their answers.
      6. Read each of the two role playing vignettes one at a time asking for volunteers for each role.
         a. After the first round of role playing, ask players to identify how each player was behaving (passively, assertively, or aggressively) and why.
         b. Have the same players switch behaviors so they can learn to act out all three in the same situation.
         c. Players may switch roles, for example, from smoker to nonsmoker.
         d. New players may try the same vignette with different responses.
      7. Have members read aloud their answers to the "personal questions."
         a. For question 2, have the group problem solve ways to act more assertively for each group member's current situation.

B. *Homework*:
   Using the group's feedback, each client will try to act more assertively in their identified current situations from personal question 2. They will discuss their progress in next session.

*Modified with permission from Schwimmer-Stern, P. Life Skills Curriculum (unpublished master's project), 1986.

Form 4-8

Assertiveness Training

One of the ways to manage stress is to be able to say what you feel, state what you need, set limits, and be able to say "no" to people, places, and things. If you can do these things, you are being assertive.

Today, we are going to train you how to be more assertive in your daily lives. The more you practice these techniques on your own, the easier they will become. In the future, they will come more naturally and you may experience less stress.

Definitions:

1. Passive—to not express your needs.
2. Assertive—to express your needs in a manner which *does not* hurt anyone emotionally or physically.
3. Aggressive—to express your needs in a manner which *does* hurt someone's feelings or hurt them physically.

Fill in the blanks:

1. If I screamed at my mother because she is always nagging me about putting my clothes away, I was acting ______________________.
   She was being ______________________ towards me.
2. When my boss gave me too much work to do and I took it anyway, I was being ______________________ .
3. When another member in the Program tried to persuade me to use drugs with him, but I said "no thanks," I was being ______________________ .

Role play:

1. You are watching a movie in a nonsmoking theater. The person next to you lights up a cigarette. The smoke bothers you. What happens next?
   a. Role players required:
      1. Smoker.
      2. Nonsmoker.
2. You are in a session with your therapist. You feel you have gotten all you can get out of the Program, but you are afraid to leave. Your therapist hands you your schedule for the next four months. Your therapist asks you how you like your new schedule.
   You respond ______________________ .
   a. Role players required:
      1. Therapist.
      2. Another member.

Personal questions:

1. In general, do you tend to be passive, assertive, or aggressive?

2. Identify a current situation where you would like to act more assertively.

SOCIAL SKILLS

Day________________

Group Leader Plan

Giving and Receiving Feedback*

I. *Objectives*: Members will be able to:
   A. Define "feedback."
   B. Understand how feedback is not criticism and how we use it in each session (reality testing, feeling of universality, encouragement, etc.)
   C. Increase the amount of feedback they give to other group members based on their own life experiences.
   D. Learn how to use feedback given to them in group, in therapy sessions, or from friends/family members in a constructive way.

II. *Materials*: Form 4-9 cut into individual squares.

III. *Procedures*:
   A. Have members define "feedback." Discuss how feedback is different from criticism.
   B. Perform the feedback therapeutic exercise.
      1. Hand out one index card at a time (cut from Form 4-9).
      2. Have a member read the card aloud and give it to another member who matches the description on the card. Ask the first member to give an example of how the second member matches that feedback.
      3. The member receiving the feedback discusses their reaction.
      4. Finish the pile in this manner.
   C. Discuss how feedback is helpful in group sessions, encouraging members to increase the amount of feedback they give.
   D. Discuss how members can use feedback they get from family, friends, therapists, or group sessions in a goal-directed way.
   E. Discuss how important feedback is for recovery.
      1. People with substance abuse go through a phase or phases of denial. Feedback from others is needed to help break the denial.
      2. Substance abuse is a sneaky, relentless disease which often tries to distort a person's judgment. People will often lie to themselves and others in the pursuit of drugs and/or alcohol. Feedback from others is necessary for reality testing.
      3. The first step is to admit powerlessness over the disease. People and their feedback are then needed for help and support through the recovery process.

*Modified from Bond, T. *Games for Life and Social Skills.* London: Hutchinson and Co., 1986, pp. 179–181.

Form 4-9

Feedback Cards

A self-destructive person	A person who loses their temper easily
A sad person	A quiet person
Someone who is using	A calm person
Someone with good hygiene	An impulsive person
An honest person	Someone who feels entitled
Someone in denial about their recovery	A person involved in risky behavior

A brave person	A person who is easy to talk to
A humorous person	A person who has trouble concentrating
A kind person	An affectionate person
A person you would like to get to know better	A person who tries hard
A person who gossips a lot	A considerate person
The person with the most clean time	The person with the most expressive face

SOCIAL SKILLS

Day__________________

Group Leader Plan

Affection

I. *Objectives*: Members will be able to:
   A. Begin to discuss their feelings about being close to people.
   B. State past experiences where they were close to someone and it felt very good.
   C. Discuss how drugs and alcohol have affected their ability to trust.
   D. Express why it is difficult to get close to people now.
   E. List different appropriate ways to receive and give affection.
   F. State how they would like to get affection.

II. *Materials*: Blackboard and chalk.

III. *Procedures*:
   A. Verbally discuss the objectives above.
      1. Leader provides a safe, supportive atmosphere in which to discuss affection as above.

SOCIAL SKILLS

Day ________________

Group Leader Plan

Making and Keeping New Friends

I. *Objectives*: Members will be able to:
   A. Identify characteristics they would *like* to have in a friend.
   B. Identify characteristics they would *not like* to have in a friend.
   C. Identify characteristics they possess that would make them a good friend.
   D. Identify what keeps them from making friends now.
   E. Problem solve around the issues in D.

II. *Materials*: Form 4-10 and pens.

III. *Procedures*:
   A. Form 4-10, "Making and Keeping New Friends."
      1. Distribute.
      2. Have members read it aloud.
      3. Explain purpose of handout.
      4. Any questions?
      5. Allow time for completion
      6. Discuss their answers.
      7. Problem solve around question 4.

Form 4-10

Making and Keeping New Friends

1. What kind of characteristics would you like to have in a friend?

2. What kind of characteristics would you *not* like your friend to have?

3. What characteristics do *you* have that would make you a good friend?

4. Why do you not have friends now?

SOCIAL SKILLS

Day____________________

Group Leader Plan

Public Speaking

I. *Objectives*: Members will be able to demonstrate and practice the following public speaking skills:
   A. Appropriate voice level.
   B. Appropriate gestures and body language.
   C. Visual cue observations.
   D. Active listening.
   E. Paraphrasing.
   F. Clarification.
   G. Organization.
   H. Delivering information in a logical, coherent manner.
   I. Speaking clearly.

II. *Materials*: Members are to bring in an object that they will base their verbal presentations on.

III. *Procedures*:
   A. Members should be informed in the session before this one to prepare a verbal presentation around a significant object that they can bring to the group.
   B. Each presentation should be approximately seven minutes.
   C. Review the objectives above before anyone speaks.
   D. After each speech, have the group give feedback about the member's public speaking skills.

REFERENCES

1. Liberman, R. P. *Social and Independent Living Skills: Basic Conversation Skills Module*. Los Angeles: Clinical Research Center for Schizophrenia and Psychiatric Rehabilitation, 1990, p. 61.

5 Activities of Daily Living for Abstinence

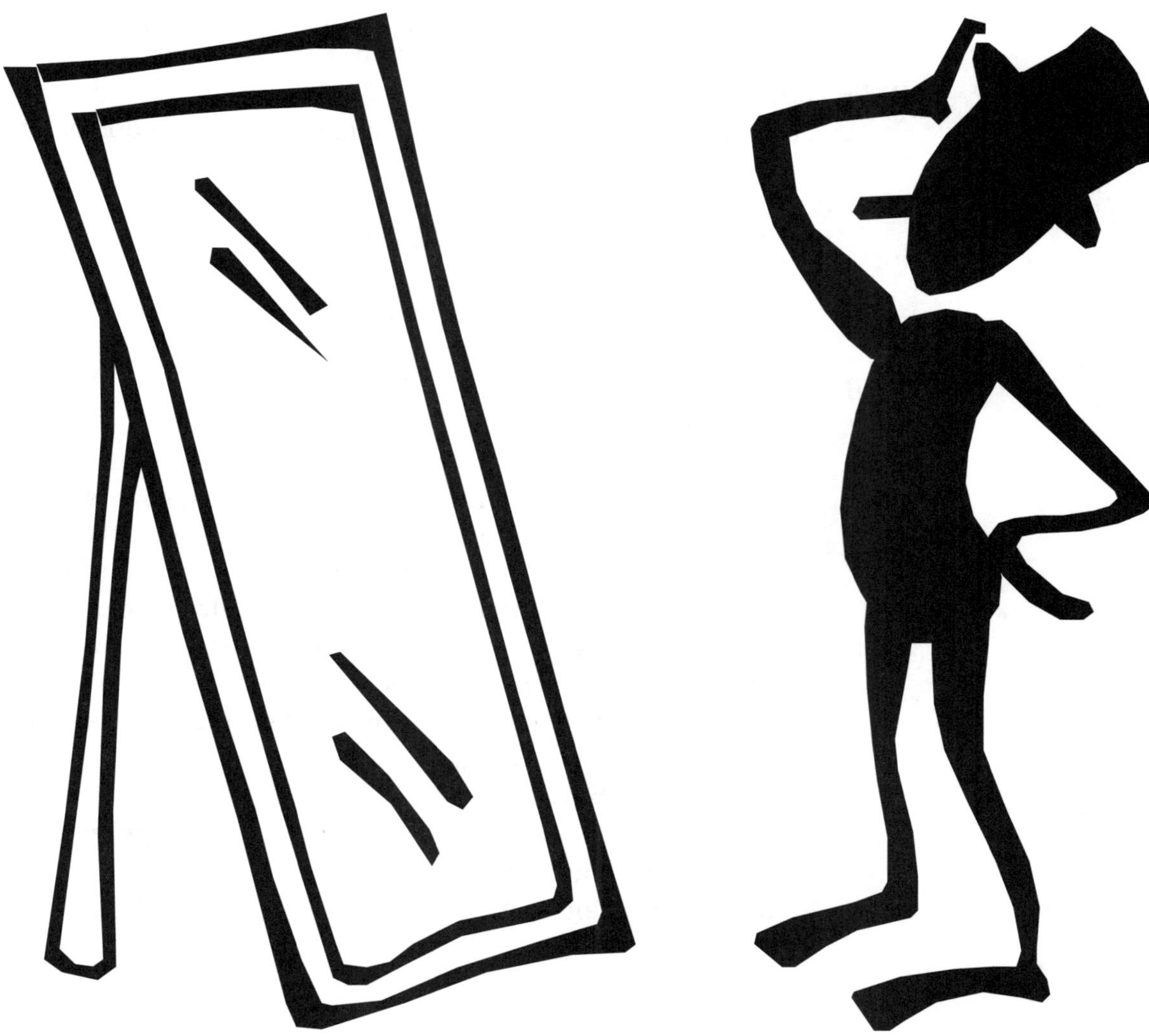

ACTIVITIES OF DAILY LIVING

Day__________________

Group Leader Plan

Activities of Daily Living (ADL) Strengths and Problems Areas

I. *Objectives*: Members will be able to:
   A. Identify some of their ADL strengths.
   B. Identify some of their ADL deficits.
   C. Identify the deficits they will try to improve during this group.
   D. Increase their understanding of why it is important for them to strengthen their ADL skills given their dual diagnoses.

II. *Materials*: Form 5-1, Form 5-2, and pens.

III. *Procedures*:
   A. Form 5-1, "Activities of Daily Living: Strengths and Problem Areas."
      1. Distribute.
      2. Have members read it aloud.
      3. Any questions?
      4. Allow time for completion.
      5. Discuss their answers.
   B. Form 5-2, "Activities of Daily Living Puzzle."
      1. Distribute
      2. Have members read the words at the top aloud.
      3. Explain the following directions to the members.
         a. Members are to search for the words listed at the top of the page in the puzzles below. Words can be formed upside down, right side up, horizontally, vertically, etc.
         b. Once a word is located, members should circle the word and cross it off the list above.
         c. Members continue in this manner until all the words have been located.
      4. Any questions?
      5. If time allows, members may begin during group time and finish at home.
      6. Review their answers in the next group session.

Activities of Daily Living: Strengths and Problem Areas

We will be spending the next sessions talking about some of the ADL skills which are necessary and important to you.

Some activities of daily living are automatic. We can do them without much thought or effort because we have done them throughout our lives, for example, going to the bathroom and walking down the street. However, other activities may be more difficult for us, like using the subway system or working.

Drugs and alcohol can get in the way of how you perform daily activities. Some people stop:

1. Showering.
2. Eating regularly.
3. Shaving.
4. Saving money.
5. Calling their friends.

Why?

Psychiatric symptoms can also affect activities of daily living. When psychiatric symptoms are bad, some people find it harder to:

1. Get up in the morning.
2. Do their laundry.
3. Clean their apartment.
4. Take care of themselves.

Why?

Keeping in mind all of the activities of daily living we have talked about so far:

1. Which ones are you good at?

2. Which ones are you *not* good at?

3. Which ones would you like to work on in this group?

Activities of Daily Living Puzzle

- Apartment
- Money Management
- Toothpaste
- Hygiene
- Bathing
- Trains
- Nutrition
- Laundry
- Pizza
- Transportation
- Subway
- Tokens
- Pots and Pans
- Beautiful
- Comb
- Brush
- Sausages
- Maintenance

M	B	Z	B	R	U	S	H	Q	U	E	S	T	Q
O	M	S	A	L	P	I	Z	Z	A	C	R	A	U
N	O	I	T	A	T	R	O	P	S	N	A	R	T
E	C	V	H	U	P	E	A	U	U	A	G	A	B
Y	W	T	I	N	C	P	B	T	U	N	T	R	M
M	U	H	N	D	O	W	R	M	I	E	B	U	S
A	S	Y	G	R	A	I	S	S	P	T	C	T	N
N	E	G	P	Y	T	N	S	I	P	N	E	O	I
A	G	I	P	I	N	E	E	A	F	I	A	K	A
G	A	E	O	M	R	F	G	H	I	A	J	E	R
E	S	N	E	D	A	P	A	R	T	M	E	N	T
M	U	E	B	E	A	U	T	I	F	U	L	S	A
E	A	I	O	J	E	P	E	S	M	D	T	I	E
N	S	R	S	N	A	P	D	N	A	S	T	O	P
T	O	O	T	H	P	A	S	T	E	T	O	L	C

ACTIVITIES OF DAILY LIVING

Day__________________

Group Leader Plan

Proper Nutrition

I. *Objectives*: Members will be able to:
   A. Eat nutritiously.
   B. Learn about vitamins, minerals, pyramid theory, fat, cholesterol, sugars, caffeine, salt, calories, low blood sugar, high blood sugar, high blood pressure.
   C. State how certain foods can affect their level of alertness.
   D. Identify their own target body weight.

II. *Materials*: Figure 5-1, Table 5-1, Table 5-2, Table 5-3, and chalk.

III. *Procedures*:
   A. Introduce how nutrition affects: mood, level of alertness, and energy levels.
   B. Emphasize the need to eat three balanced meals per day at regular intervals to maximize alertness, energy levels, and mood.
   C. Discuss the pyramid theory using Figure 5-1, "The Food Pyramid."
      1. Distribute.
      2. Have members read it aloud.
      3. Discuss how most of the daily calories should come from food items at the large base of the pyramid. As one moves up the pyramid, the amount of calories consumed from the items should be fewer and fewer. The least amount of calories consumed should be from fat, salt, and sugar shown at the tip of the pyramid.
      4. Ask members which section of the pyramid most of their calories come from.
   D. Define "calories," and briefly teach that food breaks down into energy for the body to use.
   E. Discuss that some foods give off better energy than others; fat vs. complex carbohydrates vs. simple sugars.
   F. Discuss vitamins using Table 5-1, "Vitamins."
   G. Discuss undesirable foods and drinks and why they are harmful:
      1. Fat, cholesterol, sugar, caffeine, and salt.
      2. Table 5-2, "Caffeine Counter."
         a. Distribute.
         b. Have members add up how many milligrams (mg.) of caffeine they have every day.
         c. Discuss the reasons members like to drink a lot of caffeine.
         d. Discuss other alternatives to caffeine.

H. Discuss healthy body weights.
   1. Table 5-3, "Healthy Weights for Men and Women."
      a. Distribute.
      b. Explain the set-up of the table.
      c. Have members locate their height and gender on the table to find their healthy weight range.
      d. Have members state whether or not their weight is below the range, above the range, or within the range.

Figure 5-1 The Food Pyramid

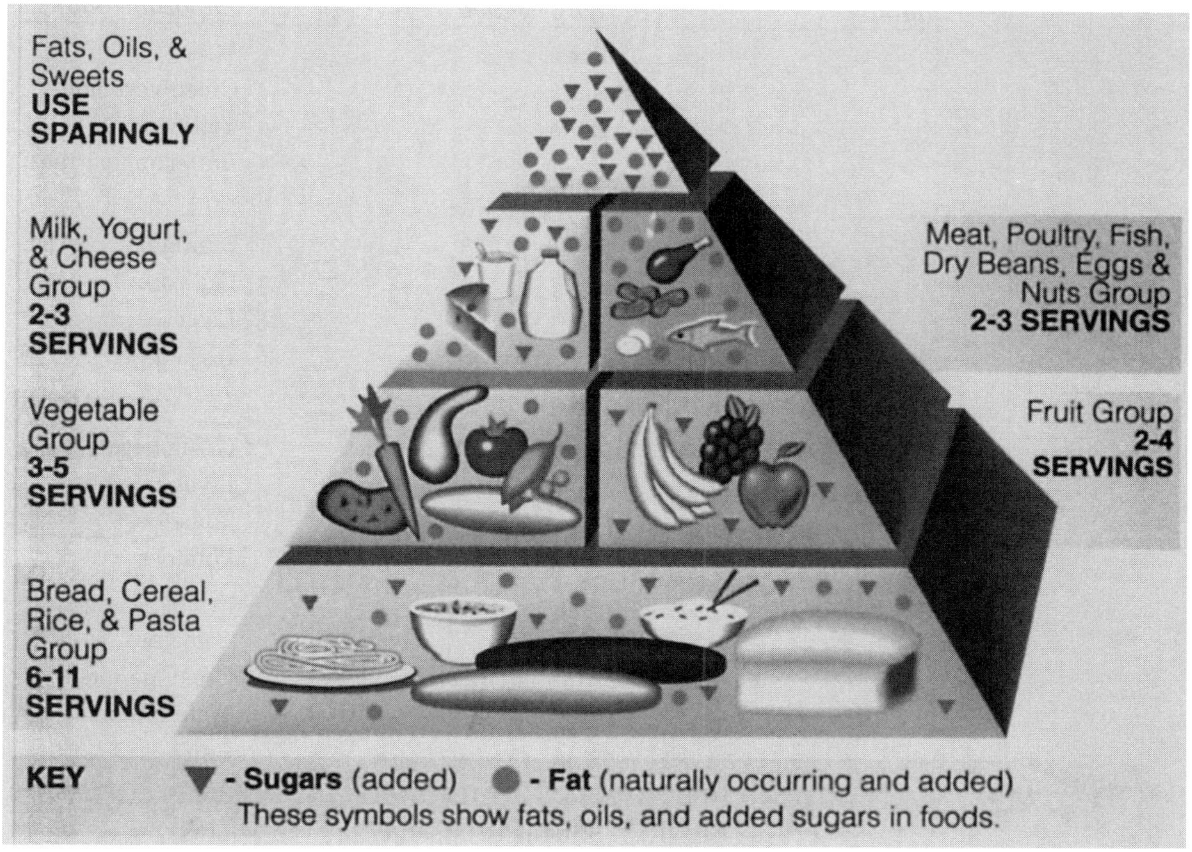

Source: U.S. Department of Agriculture.

Table 5-1 Vitamins

Vitamin	*Why needed*	*Important sources*
A	Eyes Skin Bones	Milk Green vegetables Yellow fruits Butter/margarine
D	Normal growth Bones	Milk Sunlight Egg yolk Liver
E	Antioxidant Skin	Vegetables
K	Blood clotting	Green vegetables Liver Tomatoes Potatoes
C	Bones Wounds Antioxidant Prevents colds	Fruits Tomatoes Green peppers Watermelon
B (1, 2, 3, 6, and 12)	Skin Blood Stimulates appetite	Milk Pork Liver Bread Cereals Pasta Fish

Table 5-2 Caffeine Counter

Beverage	*Serving*	*Caffeine*
Regular brewed coffee	8 oz.	100–150 mg.[1]
Decaffeinated brewed coffee	8 oz.	2–4 mg.[1]
Instant coffee	8 oz.	86–99 mg.[1]
Brewed tea	8 oz.	17–110 mg.[1, 2, 3]
Cola drinks	12 oz.	40–60 mg.[4]

Table 5-3 Healthy Weights for Men and Women

Height	*Men*	*Women*
4'10"		91–199 lbs.
4'11"		92–122 lbs.
5'0"		96–125 lbs.
5'1"		99–128 lbs.
5'2"	112–141 lbs.	102–131 lbs.
5'3"	115–144 lbs.	105–134 lbs.
5'4"	118–148 lbs.	108–138 lbs.
5'5"	121–152 lbs.	111–142 lbs.
5'6"	124–156 lbs.	114–146 lbs.
5'7"	128–161 lbs.	118–150 lbs.
5'8"	132–166 lbs.	122–154 lbs.
5'9"	136–170 lbs.	126–158 lbs.
5'10"	140–174 lbs.	130–163 lbs.
5'11"	144–179 lbs.	134–168 lbs.
6'0"	148–184 lbs.	138–173 lbs.
6'1"	152-189 lbs.	
6'2"	156-194 lbs.	
6'3"	160-199 lbs.	
6'4"	164-204 lbs.	

Source: U.S. Department of Health, Education, and Welfare.

ACTIVITIES OF DAILY LIVING

Day ____________________

Group Leader Plan

How Drugs and Alcohol Affect Nutrition

I. *Objectives*: Members will be able to:
   A. State two effects that drugs and alcohol have on their nutrition and health.
   B. State a physical sign of poor nutrition caused by drug abuse.
   C. State a physical sign of poor nutrition caused by alcohol abuse.
   D. Identify their own physical signs of poor nutrition caused by drugs/alcohol.

II. *Materials*: Blackboard and chalk.

III. *Procedures*:
   A. Teach the effects of various drugs on nutrition, using the Group Leader Plan, "Effects of Drugs on Nutrition."
   B. Teach the physical signs of poor nutrition caused by drug abuse using Group Leader Plan, "Effects of Drugs on Nutrition."
   C. Teach the effects of alcohol on nutrition using the Group Leader Plan, "Effects of Alcohol on Nutrition."
   D. Teach the physical signs of poor nutrition caused by alcohol abuse using the Group Leader Plan, "Effects of Alcohol on Nutrition."
   E. Have members identify which of the physical symptoms above they have experienced from poor nutritional habits as a result of drug/alcohol abuse. List them on the board.

ACTIVITIES OF DAILY LIVING

Day____________________

Group Leader Plan

Effects of Drugs on Nutrition

1. Stimulants may increase metabolism to the point where food is processed so quickly that vital nutrients pass right through before they can be absorbed.
2. Stimulants tend to curb appetites. That is why they are sometimes used in diet pills. However, with decreased food intake comes decreased energy from lack of vitamins and minerals.
3. Stimulants deplete potassium and magnesium very quickly. The result is feeling tired after use of stimulants because your muscles do not have enough of these to operate effectively.
4. Marijuana stimulates the appetite but not the motivation to cook healthy food. Therefore, people who are using marijuana often eat fast and easy food such as potato chips, candy, and popcorn. Over time, this can lead to malnutrition.
5. Drugs may cause cancers of the tongue, mouth, pharynx, and esophagus.[5] They may also cause digestive system problems such as ulcers, pancreatitis and gastritis.[5]

Psychological Effects of Drugs on Nutrition

People abusing substances become preoccupied with where and how to get those drugs. Most of their time is spent in this pursuit. There is less time for overall care of themselves, including eating properly. Their motivation to take care of themselves and eat properly takes second place to securing new drugs. Money for food is usually used for drugs/alcohol instead of nutritious food.

Physical Signs of Poor Nutrition Caused by Drugs

1. Pale skin from anemia caused by lack of iron.
2. Flaky, dry skin from lack of vitamin E.
3. Shrunken, dry lips from dehydration.
4. Thin body from malnutrition.[5]
5. New hair growth is lighter in color from malnutrition. Often a person's hair will have colored layers from periods of malnutrition followed by periods of adequate food intake. Hair may be brittle and dry from lack of calcium.
6. Fingernails and toenails may be yellow, brittle, appear streaked and/or contain ridges due to lack of calcium.
7. Poor dental hygiene or loss of teeth.[5]

ACTIVITIES OF DAILY LIVING

Day ____________________

Group Leader Plan

Effects of Alcohol on Nutrition

1. Alcohol has many calories with little nutritional value.[6] These are called "empty calories." People who drink a lot of alcohol feel full and eat less food. Alcoholics are typically deficient in vitamins B12 and B6, resulting in rickets and/or fatigue.
2. Alcohol is a diuretic, which means it causes the body to excrete fluids. Long-term dehydration, called *precipitous dehydration*, can result in several problems:
   a. With the loss of body fluids, the blood thickens and the heart has to work harder.
   b. Over time the heart enlarges in order to be able to pump enough "thick" blood through the body.
   c. Over time, an enlarged, overworked heart can lead to heart failure and death, usually within two years after diagnosis. [7]
3. Alcohol acts like a poison to the liver. Over time, cirrhosis of the liver can develop and lead to death.[8]

Psychological Effects of Alcohol on Nutrition
(See "Psychological Effects of Drugs on Nutrition" in previous group leader plan.)

Physical Signs of Alcohol Abuse

- Weight gain from high caloric content.[5]
- Red veins in eyes from high blood pressure. These may burst and cause blindness.[9]
- Yellow tint of skin (jaundice) from cirrhosis of liver.[8]
- Wide-based gait from poor balance due to peripheral neuropathy (the deadening of the nerves in the feet and hands) and intoxication.
- Loss of gustatory sensation. Alcohol deadens the taste buds over time.
- Many people suffering from alcoholism eat very spicy foods in order to taste their food.

ACTIVITIES OF DAILY LIVING

Day____________________

Group Leader Plan

Your Current Diet

I. *Objectives*: Members will be able to:
   A. State why it is necessary to keep track of eating habits.
   B. Use a dietary record to keep track of their eating habits.
   C. Keep a personal dietary record for at least three days during the week.

II. *Materials*: Blackboard, chalk, Form 5-3, and pens.

III. *Procedures*:
   A. Form 5-3, "My Dietary Record."
      1. Distribute.
      2. Have members fill in what they have eaten today.
      3. Discuss their answers.
      4. Introduce the importance of keeping a dietary record:
         a. To identify eating habits that are unhealthy.
         b. To relate eating habits to behavior, such as inability to concentrate, low energy levels, or cravings.
         c. To be more aware of eating habits.
         d. To adjust a diet when necessary to maintain health and sobriety.
   B. *Homework*:
      Complete Form 5-3, "My Dietary Record," for today and two other days during the week. Discuss results during next two sessions.

Form 5-3

My Dietary Record

Date ______________________

Breakfast

Amount	*Food*	*Food Group*	*Calories*	*Vitamins*

Lunch

Amount	*Food*	*Food Group*	*Calories*	*Vitamins*

Dinner

Amount	*Food*	*Food Group*	*Calories*	*Vitamins*

Snack

Amount	*Food*	*Food Group*	*Calories*	*Vitamins*

ACTIVITIES OF DAILY LIVING

Day____________________

Group Leader Plan

Positive Dietary Goals

I. *Objectives*: Members will be able to:
   A. Review their "Dietary Records" and identify their nutritional problem areas.
   B. Write short-term goals to address their identified problem areas.
   C. Describe why their goal is important to them.
   D. List possible steps to achieve their goal.
   E. Perform the steps by next week.
   F. Report progress back to the group.
   G. Make improvements in their diets.

II. *Materials*: Form 5-3, blackboard, chalk, and pens.

III. *Procedures*:
   A. Form 5-3, "My Dietary Record."
      1. Have members review their "Dietary Records" and identify at least one problem area in their diets (from last session's Form 5-3, "My Dietary Record").
   B. Appendix 1, Form A1-3, "Goal Setting Worksheet."
      1. Distribute.
      2. Have members read it aloud.
      3. Any questions?
      4. Allow time for completion.
      5. Discuss their answers.
   C. *Homework*:
      Members will follow through on their positive dietary goals and report their progress next session.

ACTIVITIES OF DAILY LIVING

Day__________________

Group Leader Plan

Hygiene and Grooming

I. *Objectives*: Members will be able to:
   A. List a variety of hygiene and grooming activities.
   B. Discuss why hygiene and grooming are important activities of daily living.
   C. Understand that cultural and social influences affect hygiene and grooming practices.
   D. List how often they perform certain hygiene and grooming activities.
   E. Determine their strengths and problem areas with regard to hygiene and grooming.

II. *Materials*: Group Leader Plan, "Hygiene Activity Sheet," Form 5-4, blackboard, chalk, and pens.

III. *Procedures*:
   A. Introduce topic by defining hygiene and grooming.
   B. Have members call out all of the hygiene and grooming activities they can think of, and write them on the board. Fill in what they missed using the group leader plan "Hygiene Activity Sheet."
   C. Form 5-4, "My Personal Hygiene and Grooming."
      1. Distribute.
      2. Have members read it aloud.
      3. Any questions?
      4. Allow time for completion.
      5. Discuss their answers.

My Personal Hygiene and Grooming

List how often you do the following activities:

Shower/bathe:

Brush teeth:

Floss teeth:

Wash face:

Shave or trim beard or mustache:

Apply deodorant:

Wash hands:

Wash hair:

Comb/style hair:

Clean under nails (fingers and toes):

Trim and file nails (fingers and toes):

Change underwear:

Change clothes:

Clean ears:

What areas do you think you are good at?

What areas do you think you have problems with?

ACTIVITIES OF DAILY LIVING

Day ____________________

Group Leader Plan

Hygiene Activity Sheet

1. Hygiene Activities
   - using mouthwash
   - brushing teeth
   - brushing hair
   - shaving
   - trimming mustache and beard
   - changing underwear
   - changing clothes
   - using moisturizer for lips
   - using appropriate amount of cologne or after shave
   - cleaning ears
   - clearing corners of eyes
   - applying deodorant
   - using powder
   - cleaning under nails and keeping nails at an appropriate length, including toenails
   - caring for eyeglasses
   - bathing
   - keeping rectum and genitals clean
   - washing hands after using the bathroom
   - washing hands before and after eating
   - purchasing grooming and hygiene products
   - keeping towels clean and dry
2. Other Considerations
   - Cleanliness for one person may be different than for others.
   - Hygiene habits are affected by culture and social influences.
   - Lack of personal hygiene may be the first indication of emotional problems and/or substance abuse.
   - How does one decide when to wash?
3. Why is hygiene important?
   - Health (prevent disease and infection).
   - Social acceptability (people who emit strong body odor may be ostracized).
   - Necessary for jobs, interviews, and volunteer positions.
   - Helps people feel better.
   - Helps people have more friends.

ACTIVITIES OF DAILY LIVING

Day_________________

Group Leader Plan

Effects of Drugs and Alcohol on Hygiene and Grooming

I. *Objectives*: Members will be able to:
   A. List the various effects that drugs and alcohol have on their hygiene and grooming.
   B. List the physical signs of poor grooming and hygiene that are caused by alcohol and substance abuse.
   C. Discuss ways in which their alcohol/substance abuse has affected their hygiene and grooming.

II. *Materials*: Blackboard and chalk.

III. *Procedures*:
   A. Have members call out ways in which alcohol and drugs affect hygiene and grooming.
   B. Write answers on the board.
   C. Discuss the physical signs of the problems listed above (such as yellow teeth, brittle hair, cracked fingernails, bloodshot eyes).
   D. Have members discuss their own experiences with hygiene and grooming problems caused by alcohol and/or drug abuse.

ACTIVITIES OF DAILY LIVING

Day____________________

Group Leader Plan

Identifying Current Monthly Expenses

I. *Objectives*: Members will be able to:
   A. Generate examples of monthly expenses.
   B. Identify their current monthly expenses.
   C. Total their current monthly expenses.
   D. State how drugs/alcohol may be affecting their current expenses.
II. *Materials*: Form 5-5, Form 5-6, blackboard, chalk, and pens.
III. *Procedures*:
   A. Introduce topic of budgeting by discussing awareness of monthly expenses.
   B. Form 5-5, "Possible Expenses."
      1. Distribute.
      2. Have members read it aloud.
      3. Any questions?
      4. Allow time for completion.
      5. Discuss their answers.
      6. Write their answers on the board and add items as needed.
   C. Form 5-6, "Identifying My Current Expenses."
      1. Distribute.
      2. Have members list which expenses they *currently* have. They may refer to the answers in Form 5-5, "Possible Expenses."
      3. Have members estimate, as closely as possible, how much they spend on each item they listed.
      4. Have members add up total monthly expenses.
      5. If possible, have members subtract total monthly expenses from total income.
      6. Discuss results.
      7. Discuss how drugs/alcohol may be affecting their current expenses.

Possible Expenses

List below possible monthly expenses. They may be expenses that you currently have, expenses you had in the past, or expenses you know that other people have.

Form 5-6

Identifying My Current Expenses

List your current monthly expenses.

ITEM	*AMOUNT SPENT*
	TOTAL $ SPENT EACH MONTH

ACTIVITIES OF DAILY LIVING

Day____________________

Group Leader Plan

Identifying Fixed versus Flexible Expenses*

I. *Objectives*: Members will be able to:
   A. Define a "budget."
   B. Define "fixed" and "flexible" expenses and tell how they are different.
   C. Classify their current expenses as either fixed or flexible.
   D. Discuss ways in which flexible expenses may be cut or even increased, as needed.

II. *Materials*: Form 5-7, Form 5-8, Form 5-9, blackboard, chalk, and pens.

III. *Procedures*:
   A. Define "budget" as "a plan that allows you to coordinate your resources and your expenses."
   B. Discuss definition.
   C. Define "fixed expenses" as "expenses that never vary or rarely vary."
   D. Discuss definition and examples.
   E. Define "flexible expenses" as "expenses that vary quite often."
   F. Discuss definition and examples.
   G. Form 5-6, "Identifying My Current Expenses," which was given out and used during last session.
      1. Have members indicate next to each previously identified expense, whether it is fixed or flexible.
   H. Form 5-7, "My Expenses."
      1. Distribute.
      2. Have members read it aloud.
      3. Have members list their fixed and flexible expenses (they may refer to Form 5-6, "Identifying My Current Expenses").
      4. Have members discuss their individual fixed and flexible expenses and how they may want to change their current flexible expenses.
      5. Have members write short-term goals to actualize their desired changes.
   I. Form 5-8, "Resources."
      1. Distribute.
      2. Have members read it aloud.
      3. Any questions?
      4. Allow time for completion.
      5. Discuss their answers.

J. Form 5-9, "Summary."
1. Distribute.
2. Have members read it aloud.
3. Any questions?
4. Allow time for completion.
5. Discuss their answers.

*Modified with permission from Schwimmer-Stern, P. Life Skills Curriculum (unpublished master's project), 1986.

My Expenses

"Fixed" monthly expenses are expenses that stay the same every month (like rent). "Flexible" monthly expenses are expenses that change every month (like buying a pair of shoes once a year). List both below in the appropriate column.

Fixed Monthly Expense		Flexible Expense	
Expense	Amount	Expense	Amount
Total +	________	Total +	________
Fixed Expenses =	$________	Flexible Expenses =	$________

$________ Total Monthly Expenses

Form 5-8

Resources

A "Fixed" monthly resource is a certain amount of money that comes to you every month throughout the year, for example, social security income or disability.

A "Flexible" resource is an amount of money that you receive just one time or inconsistently throughout the year (like a gift).

Please list your money sources below.

Fixed Monthly Resources		Flexible Resources	
Source	Amount	Source	Amount
	+ ______		+ ______
	= $______		= $______

$______ Total Monthly Resources

Summary

My total monthly resources minus
My total monthly expenses = $ __________

This is how much money I have left over at the end of the month.
If it is less than zero, I have overspent and need to

BUDGET

If it is less than what I would like, I need to

BUDGET

If I am not happy with the way I spend money, I need to

BUDGET

Do I need to budget? __________ Yes __________ No

ACTIVITIES OF DAILY LIVING

Day__________________

Group Leader Plan

My Budget Plan

I. *Objectives*: Members will be able to:
   A. Make a budget for themselves for the following month using newly learned money management skills to correct problems they have had in the past.
   B. Identify which expenses they have to cut down on.
   C. Begin to follow this budget.
   D. Discuss and note any difficulties in sticking to their new budget.

II. *Materials*: Form 5-10 and pens.

III. *Procedures*:
   A. Form 5-10, "My New Budget."
      1. Distribute.
      2. Have members read it aloud.
      3. Any questions?
      4. Allow time for completion.
      5. Discuss their answers.

My New Budget

For the month of ______________________________ .
I will limit my expenses to:

Expense	Amount
Total	+ ________ $

I will cut down on the following:

ACTIVITIES OF DAILY LIVING

Day ____________________

Group Leader Plan

Decision Making*

I. *Objectives*: Members will be able to:
   A. Identify and prioritize a current decision that they need to make.
   B. List the pros and cons.
   C. Weigh the pros and cons.
   D. List any steps that they could take to help them make an educated decision.
   E. Modify the decision if necessary.
   F. Commit to the decision, carry it out, and discuss the results.
   G. Take more responsibility for their actions.
   H. Maximize their sense of control.
   I. Increase their judgment.
   J. Increase independent functioning in their environment.

II. *Materials*: Form 5-11 and pens.

III. *Procedures*:
   A. Form 5-11, "Recovery and Decision Making Worksheet."
      1. Distribute.
      2. Have members read it aloud.
      3. Discuss.
         a. Ask members which of them has ever been impulsive.
         b. Encourage members to give examples of how they acted impulsively.
      4. Allow time for completion.
      5. Discuss their answers.
   B. *Homework*:
      1. Have each member carry out some aspect of or all of their decision.
      2. Have them report results next session.

*Modified with permission from Korb, K. L., Azok, S., and Leutenberg, E. A. *Life Management Skills I.* Beachwood, OH: Wellness Reproductions, Inc., 1993, p. 25.

Recovery and Decision Making Worksheet

People with substance abuse problems sometimes act without thinking things through first. This is called being impulsive. The result may be doing things that they regret or getting themselves into trouble. Here is an easy exercise to help you think through a decision, so you can make an educated choice. To do this, you need to see both sides of the coin, the positive and the negative, before you decide. Hopefully, you will be happier about you decisions. Making choices will no longer be overwhelming, and it will be easier to keep your clean time.

I would like to decide whether or not to:

____

____

Pros	*Cons*
1.	1.
2.	2.
3.	3.
4.	4.
5.	5.
6.	6.

My decision is to:

____

____

ACTIVITIES OF DAILY LIVING

Day__________________

Group Leader Plan

Introduction to Exercise

I. *Objectives*: Members will be able to:
   A. List some of the benefits of exercise.
   B. Identify what types of exercise they may enjoy.
   C. Set an exercise goal for themselves and follow through with it.

II. *Materials*: Group Leader Plan "The Many Benefits of Exercise," Form 5-12, Form 5-13, Table 5-4, blackboard, chalk, and pens.

III. *Procedures*:
   A. Form 5-12, "The Many Benefits of Exercise."
      1. Distribute.
      2. Have members read it aloud.
      3. Discuss each benefit one by one beginning with "psychological," "cardiovascular," and so forth.
         a. Define the benefit.
         b. Have members call out as many benefits under that heading as they can.
         c. Record their answers on the board.
         d. Have members take notes on their form.
         e. Add any benefits they missed using your group leader plan "The Many Benefits of Exercise."
         f. Pause in between responses and ask members for examples of personal experiences.
   B. Form 5-13, "Deciding What Kind of Exercise Is Right for Me."
      1. Distribute.
      2. Have members read it aloud.
      3. Any questions?
      4. Allow time for completion.
      5. Discuss their answers.
   C. Table 5-4, "Benefits of Sports."
      1. Distribute.
      2. Define "cardiac, muscle endurance, muscle strength, coordination, balance, and flexibility," giving demonstrations of each.
      3. Have members discuss which of these sports they have participated in before, describe what the sport was like and state any positive experiences derived from it.

4. Have members circle one sport they would like to pursue in the future based on the sport's benefits and based on their own needs from Form 5-13, "Deciding What Kind of Exercise Is Right for Me."

D. *Homework*:
Have members set an exercise goal for themselves and discuss it in the following session.

ACTIVITIES OF DAILY LIVING

Day ____________________

Group Leader Plan

The Many Benefits of Exercise

1. Psychological:
   - may help people gain more control over their lives.[10]
   - improvements in perception of body image.[11]
   - more positive self-concepts.[11]
   - decrease anxiety and depression.[11]
   - increased relaxation.[10]
   - enhanced motivation.[10]
   - reduced stress.[10]
   - may decrease cravings for drugs/alcohol, caffeine, sugar, and fat.
   - keeps people away from people, places, and things.
2. Cardiovascular:
   - strengthens heart muscle.[12]
   - walls of heart become thicker and stronger, allowing it to pump more blood per beat.[12]
   - lungs increase in capacity to bring more oxygen into the system.[10]
   - can perform for longer periods of time.[10]
3. Weight Control:[10]
   - increases metabolism, which burns more calories during and after exercise.
   - lowers body fat.
   - decreases loss of muscle tissue during weight loss.
   - helps suppress appetite.
   - regulates insulin, which is responsible for guiding fat into body cells for storage.
4. Muscular:[10]
   - increases muscle efficiency.
   - increases strength.
   - increases balance.
   - increases coordination.
   - increases flexibility.
   - increases speed.
   - increases endurance.
5. Disease Prevention:
   - osteoporosis.[12, 13]
   - heart disease (exercise decreases low-density lipoproteins [LDL] and increases high-density lipoproteins [HDL]).[12]
6. Overall:[10]
   - improves sleeping habits.
   - increases energy.
   - fewer gastrointestinal disorders.
   - promotes better posture.
   - increases productivity.
   - improves appearance.
   - can be done instead of taking drugs.

The Many Benefits of Exercise

1. Psychological:

2. Cardiovascular:

3. Weight Control:

4. Muscular:

5. Disease Prevention:

6. Overall:

Form 5-13

Deciding What Kind of Exercise Is Right for Me

"One of the best motivations for physical activity is ENJOYMENT!!!"[14]

It is best when exercise does not feel like a chore or an obligation, but rather, like something fun to do. The following questions may help me determine what kind of exercises would be right for my needs.[15]

1. What are my goals?
   a. Do I want to lose weight?
   b. Do I want to maintain my current weight?
   c. Do I want to improve strength?
   d. Do I want to be more flexible?

   These are just some goals I may have. There are many more goals that exercise can help me achieve. These are some more I can think of now:

2. What are my body's capabilities?
   a. When is the last time I exercised?
   b. These are my current medical problems:
   c. These are my current physical limitations:
   d. The last time I saw my doctor for a physical exam was:
   e. Is my body ready to exercise?

3. What kind of time do I have available?
   a. Can I make time to exercise daily?
   b. Can I exercise for a few minutes at a time or do I have a few larger chunks of time to set aside?

4. Do I have money to spend on exercise?
   a. Can I buy exercise equipment?
   b. Can I buy sneakers?
   c. Can I join a gym?

5. Would I enjoy exercising alone or with others?

6. What are my personal preferences?
   a. Do I like to be outside?
   b. Am I competitive?

Table 5-4 Benefits of Sports

Sport	*Balance*	*Flexibility*	*Coordination*	*Muscle Strength*	*Muscle Endurance*	*Cardiac*
Aerobics[16]	X	X	X	X	X	X
Badminton[16]			X		X	X
Basketball[16]	X	X	X	X	X	X
Bicycling[16]	X		X		X	X
Bowling[16]	X		X	X		
Calisthenics[16]	X	X	X	X	X	X
Croquet[16]			X			
Cross-Country Skiing[16]	X		X		X	X
Darts[15]			X			
Fly Fishing[15]				X	X	X
Gardening[16]	X	X	X		X	X
Handball[16]	X	X	X	X	X	X
Hiking[16]	X			X	X	X
Housework[16]					X	X
Jogging[16]	X		X	X	X	X
Jump Rope[16]	X		X	X		X
Racquetball[16]	X	X	X	X	X	X
Rowing[16]			X	X	X	X
Skating[16]	X	X	X	X	X	X
Softball[16]			X		X	X
Soccer[16]	X	X	X	X	X	X
Stair Climbing[16]					X	X
Stationary Cycle[16]					X	X
Stretching[16]	X	X	X			
Swimming[16]		X	X	X	X	X
Table Tennis[16]			X			X
Volleyball[16]	X	X	X	X	X	X
Walking[16]						X
Weight Lifting[16]				X		

ACTIVITIES OF DAILY LIVING

Day__________________

Group Leader Plan

Review of Personal Goals

I. *Objectives*: Members will be able to:
   A. Restate their personal goals that were set throughout the Activities of Daily Living for Abstinence topic areas.
   B. State whether or not they achieved each goal.
   C. State whether or not they wish to continue each goal.
   D. Acknowledge how much progress they made during this topic area.
   E. Feel good about their progress.
   F. Begin to review course material.

II. *Materials*: Form 5-14 and pens.

III. *Procedures*:
   A. Form 5-14, "My Personal Goals."
      1. Distribute.
      2. Have members read it aloud.
      3. Any questions?
      4. Allow time for completion (members may flip through their workbooks to help them restate their goals).
      5. Discuss their answers.

My Personal Goals

During the Activities for Daily Living for Abstinence topic area, I have set the following goals:

My Nutrition Goal

____

____

Achieved: yes/no   Continue: yes/no

My Hygiene Goal

____

____

Achieved: yes/no   Continue: yes/no

My Budgeting Goal

____

____

Achieved: yes/no   Continue: yes/no

My Fitness Goal

____

____

Achieved: yes/no   Continue: yes/no

My Recovery Goal

____

____

Achieved: yes/no   Continue: yes/no

My Food Preparation Goal

____

____

Achieved: yes/no   Continue: yes/no

Other Goals I Have Set

____

____

Achieved: yes/no   Continue: yes/no

REFERENCES

1. Truitt, E. B. The Xanthines. In *Drill's Pharmacology in Medicine*, 4th ed. Edited by Dipalma, J. R. New York: McGraw-Hill, 1971, p. 547.
2. Martiner, R. G., and Wolman, W. Xanthines, tannis and sodium in coffee, tea and cocoa. *J. Amer. Med. Ass.* 158 (1955): 1030–1031.
3. Roth, J. A., Ivy, A. C., Atkinson, A. J. Caffeine and "peptic" ulcer: Relation of caffeine and caffeine-containing beverages to the pathogenesis, diagnosis and management of "peptic" ulcer. *J. Amer. Med. Ass.* 126 (1944): 814–820.
4. Greden, J. F. Coffee, tea and you. *Science* 19 (6) (1979): 9.
5. Daley, C. D., and Thase, M. E. *Dual Disorders Recovery Counseling: A Biopsychosocial Treatment Model for Addiction and Psychiatric Illness.* Independence, MO: Herald House/Independence Press, 1994, pp. 76–77.
6. Balboni, C. Alcohol in relation to dietary patterns. In Lucia, SP (ed.), *Alcohol and civilization.* New York: McGraw-Hill, 1963.
7. National Institute on Alcohol Abuse and Alcoholism. *Eighth Special Report to the U.S. Congress on Alcohol and Death.* DHSS Publication No. (ADM) 281-91-0003. Washington, DC: Public Health Service, 1993.
8. Billings, J. S., et al. *Physiological Aspects of Liquor Problems.* New York: Houghton Mifflin, 1903.
9. Ducimetiere, P., Guize, L., Marciniak, A., Milton, H., Richard, J., and Rufat, P. Arteriographically documented coronary artery disease and alcohol consumption. *European Heart Journal* 14 (b) (1993): 727–733.
10. Mullen, K. D., Gold, R. S., Belcastro, P. A., McDermott, R. J. *Connections for Health.* Dubuque: Wm C. Brown, 1986, pp. 143, 144, 148.
11. Dienstbier, R. A. The effects of exercise on personality. In Sachs, M. L., Buttore, G. W. (eds.) *Running as Therapy: An Integrated Approach.* Lincoln: Univ. of Nebraska Press, 1984, pp. 253–272.
12. McKeon, R. L. Reported by Villanueva, W. Exercise: 72 Million Americans can't be wrong—Or can they? *Discover* 3.8 (1982): 84–88; Haskel and Superko, "Exercise Plan."
13. Williams, S. R. How beneficial is regular exercise? *Journal of Cardiovascular Medicine* 7.11 (1982): 1112–1120; Villanueva, "Exercise."
14. Hunt, P., and Hillsdon, M. *Changing Eating and Exercise Behavior.* Oxford: Blackwell Science Ltd., 1996, pp. 104–107.
15. Dinabile, V. A., Levine, B., and Levitz, L. *Fitness That Fits You! A Personalized Approach to Healthy Living!* Del Rio, TX: CPC Specialty Products, Inc., 1994, p. 12.
16. American Heart Association and American Cancer Society. *Living Well: Staying Well, Big Health Rewards from Small Life Changes.* New York: Times Books, 1996, pp. 177–197.

Appendix 1: Sessions Common to All Four Topic Areas

ALL TOPICS

Group Leader Plan

Introduction

I. *Objectives*: Members will be able to:
   A. Identify the four topic areas of the workbook.
   B. Begin to understand how the workbook can help them.
II. *Materials*: Form A1-1.
III. *Procedures*:
   A. Form A1-1, "Introduction."
      1. Distribute.
      2. Have members read it aloud.
      3. Pause between paragraphs to ask for questions, comments, or life experiences related to text.
      4. Announce how the treatment will proceed.
         a. State if the treatment will take place in a group setting, one to one, or independently.
         b. State when, where, and how often the treatment will take place.
         c. State which topic will be discussed first.

Introduction

Welcome to Living Skills Recovery.

This workbook may be helpful to you if you would like to learn more about how to meet new people, how to structure your free time, and how to better cope with daily stressors. It may also be helpful to you if you suffer from substance abuse.

Having both an addiction and mental health problems can make it difficult for you to get through life and achieve your goals. But, there are certain skills which you can learn and we can teach that can help you handle situations more effectively.

This workbook focuses on four topics which dually diagnosed clients most frequently identify as troublesome. They are:

1. Time management
2. Stress management
3. Social skills
4. Activities of daily living (ADL)

Addiction and mental illness affect all of these skills. This workbook will help you identify and build your strengths in each area while also learning new material.

We believe learning should be fun, and that what you learn should be useful to your life. Therefore, there are some homework assignments, role plays, therapeutic games, and paper and pencil exercises to practice new material.

ALL TOPICS

Group Leader Plan

Defining "Time Management," "Stress Management," "Social Skills," and "Activities for Daily Living"

I. *Objectives*: Members will be able to:
   A. Define "time management," "stress management," "social skills," or "ADL."
   B. Demonstrate their current knowledge of time management, stress management, social skills, or ADL.
   C. List different components of time management, stress management, social skills, or ADL.
   D. Define the different components of the particular area to be studied.

II. *Materials*: Blackboard, chalk, and pens.

III. *Procedures*:
   A. Definitions.
      1. Ask members to define the topic area.
      2. Write correct answers on the board as they are spoken.
      3. Generate discussion around the different definitions.
      4. Generate a definition which incorporates all of the correct answers.
         a. "Time management" is the ability to regulate the way you spend your 24-hour day.
         b. "Stress management" is the skill of tolerating challenging situations so they do not become unbearable.
         c. "Social skills" is the ability to interact with others in a healthy way.
         d. "ADL" are the purposeful tasks which need to be performed every day.
      5. Generate discussion around the definitions above.
   B. Stating the different components of time management, stress management, social skills, or ADL.
      1. Ask members to list some components of time management, stress management, social skills, or ADL.
      2. Write the correct answers on the board as they are spoken.
      3. Add any components that were not mentioned (refer to the table of contents).
   C. Defining the different components of time management, stress management, social skills, or ADL.
      1. Go through each component on the board and ask members to define each one of them.
      2. Ask members for personal examples of each.

ALL TOPICS

Group Leader Plan

Goal Setting

I. *Objectives*: Members will be able to:
   A. Identify a problem related to the topic and their recovery.
   B. Set a short-term goal between now and next session that reflects their problem. Goals will be concrete, measurable, realistic, and written down.
   C. Describe why the goal is important to them.
   D. List four steps to take to achieve the goal.
   E. Perform the steps before next session.
   F. Discuss how they did with the goal in the next session. If they could not do it, what went wrong, and how could they modify it for the next time? If they were able to achieve it, how did they do it?
   G. Prioritize their goals.
   H. Understand why it is important for each goal to:
      1. Be written down.
      2. Have a deadline.
      3. Be their own, not something that someone else suggested they do.
      4. Be realistic.
      5. Be measurable.

II. *Materials*: Form A1-2, Form A1-3, and pens.

III. *Procedures*:
   A. Form A1-2, "Goal Setting."
      1. Distribute.
      2. Have members read it aloud.
      3. Stop in between paragraphs and ask for questions about the material. Do they agree or disagree with the material?
      4. Ask members to relate personal examples to each paragraph.
   B. Form A1-3, "Goal Setting Worksheet."
      1. Distribute.
      2. Have members read it aloud.
      3. Any questions?
      4. Allow time for completion.
      5. Go over each members' goals and make sure they are:
         a. Short term
         b. Measurable
         c. Concrete
         d. Realistic
         e. Reflect a problem area
         f. Steps that are solutions to the goal

6. If a member has difficulty thinking of a goal, remind them of why they are in dual diagnosis.
7. If a member has difficulty thinking of four steps, let the group help that member by problem solving from their own life experiences.
8. Emphasize that these goal setting sheets are to be taken home to remind them of what they are working on and should be brought to the next group for a discussion of their achievement.
9. Tell members that these same goal setting sheets can be used over and over again for any type of goal, and that we will use them again. Eventually, in their lives, they will not need the sheets but will have learned to set goals as a natural process.

Goal Setting

SIX POINTS TO REMEMBER*

1. Goals Should Be Written Down.

By writing down your goals, you are making a contract with yourself. You will be more likely to follow through with your goals if you put them on paper, rather than just having them in your thoughts. Writing down your goals will help you remember what you are working on. You can always refer back to your sheet of paper and note your progress. The act of writing down your goals helps you to prioritize and organize them. It can help you think more clearly about your problems so you will not be overwhelmed. Writing your goals gives you a starting point and a focus to solve your problems.

2. Your Goals Should Be Your Own.

If you set a goal for yourself, you are more likely to achieve it than if someone else tells you what to do. You can always receive and use helpful feedback from family members, therapists, or group members, but you need to have your own motivation for these suggestions in order to follow them through. It is a skill to learn how to think of steps to take to achieve your goals. So, it is useful for you to practice setting your goals yourself, because you will be the person carrying them out.

3. Goals Should Be Realistic and Attainable.

It is difficult when you set a goal too high and cannot achieve it. It can make you feel bad about yourself, like a failure. If you end up feeling this way, it is unlikely that you will want to set more goals in the future, so it is important to set realistic, achievable goals. If you are not sure how much you can do, start small and do extra if you can. This may cause you to feel a sense of accomplishment and want to practice setting more goals in the future.

4. Goals Should Be Measurable and Concrete.

It is difficult to tell if you have achieved your goal if your goal cannot be measured. For example, instead of saying that your goal is to be less anxious, how about "I will learn three new stress management techniques by next week"? Try to be as specific and concrete as you can. Instead of saying that you will do exercises, you could say "I will walk to and from the program on Monday through Friday, and will do 15 minutes of stretching exercises Sunday afternoon."

5. Work on Short-Term Goals.

In order to achieve long-term goals, like getting back to work or going to school, you have to focus on short-term goals that will help you get there. You may have a difficult time going to school if your concentration is poor or if your attendance is bad. Take one step at a time, day by day.

6. Set a Deadline for Your Goals.

Allowing yourself a specific amount of time for your goals will help you follow through with them. This will also help you avoid procrastinating or feeling overwhelmed or anxious. Dates can help you focus, and improve your motivation. They can be adjusted with changing conditions.

The Five Steps of Goal Setting:

1. Identify a problem.
2. Write a goal reflecting the problem.
3. State why the goal is important to you.
4. List four steps to achieve the goal.
5. Execute the steps.

*Modified with permission from Schwimmer-Stern, P. Life Skills Curriculum (unpublished master's project), 1986.

Form A1-3

Goal Setting Worksheet*

Set a short-term goal for yourself to be completed between (today's date) ____________ and (next session's date) ____________. The goal should be realistic, measurable, and concrete.

1. What is the problem?

2. What is your goal?

3. How is this goal important to your recovery?

4. List four steps that will help you achieve your goal between now and next session.

*Modified with permission from Hiller-Scott, A., Haggarty, E. J. Structuring goals via goal attainment scaling in occupational therapy groups in a partial hospitalization setting. *Occupational Therapy in Mental Health* 4(2) (1984): 53.

ALL TOPICS

Day__________________

Group Leader Plan

Review

I. *Objectives*: Members will be able to:
   A. State which sessions they completed and which they missed.
   B. Review each session they completed.

II. *Materials*: Blackboard, chalk, pens, and *Living Skills Recovery Workbook*.

III. *Procedures*:
   A. Identifying missing sessions.
      1. Read the title of each session one by one.
      2. After reading each aloud, ask which members completed that session.
      3. Have members note which sessions they have missed.
      4. Give positive feedback for all the sessions they have attended.
   B. Reviewing sessions.
      1. Read the first session aloud.
      2. Have members discuss what they remember about that session.
      3. If they do not remember much, they can refer back to their workbooks.
      4. Discuss what the main purpose of the session was and any other salient features they left out. Ask members for their particular goals they may have set for the session. Ask them how the goal is going at present.
      5. Repeat above for each session. This may take many sessions to review, depending on how much they recall and how much time you want to devote to a review.
      6. Remind them that they will be having a post quiz.
   C. Review the Prequiz, Form A2-2, "Stress Management Quiz," or Form A2-1, "Time Management Quiz," or Form A2-3, "Social Skills Quiz," or Form A2-4, "Activities of Daily Living Quiz." Help members go over the correct answers.
   D. *Homework*:
      Members should review their material for the postquiz.

ALL TOPICS

Day___________________

Group Leader Plan

Graduation

I. *Objectives*: Members will be able to:
   A. Receive a certificate of graduation, of perfect attendance, and/or of the number of sessions attended for each topic of the Living Skills Recovery module.
   B. Review how much progress they made in the group.
   C. Celebrate that progress with a graduation party.
   D. Discuss which new topic of the Living Skills Curriculum they will be moving on to.
   E. Build their self-esteem through completion of a topic.
   F. Terminate with group members.

II. *Materials*: Form A1-4 and Table A2-1, "Quality Assurance Data Sheet," completed ahead of time for each member, and food and party favors.

III. *Procedures*:
   A. Review members' progress.
      1. Share with members their scores recorded in Table A2-1, "Quality Assurance Data Sheet."
         a. Pretest score (% correct).
         b. Posttest score (% correct).
         c. Attendance (% of days attended).
         d. Objectives met (% of total objectives achieved).
         e. Goals met (# of goals achieved).
         f. Members report:
            1. Learned new material (check for "yes").
            2. Made changes in life (check for "yes").
         g. Staff observations—record of improvements made in social skills since the onset of the topic, for example, better related to peers, more assertive in individual sessions increased group participation.
         h. Clean time—The number of clean days since the start of the topic.
   B. Certificates.
      1. Each member should get at least one certification:
         a. Certification of Graduation if they met 70% or more of their objectives.
         b. Certification of Perfect Attendance if they achieved perfect attendance or if they completed all forms in the topic area.

c. Certification of the Number of Sessions Attended are for members who did not achieve 70% or more of the objectives and, therefore, did not graduate, but are rewarded for the number of sessions they attended—state that number on their certification. They may or may not repeat the topic.

d. Certification of Clean Time for improvements made in clean time.

C. Termination with group members.

1. Go around the room and ask people to say good-bye to each other and state which Living Skills Recovery Topic they will be covering next.

D. Graduation Party.

1. Music.
2. Food.
3. Positive feedback for all they have achieved.

____

HAS ACHIEVED

____

THROUGH THE
LIVING SKILLS RECOVERY CURRICULUM

_______________________ Signature

_____________ Date

Appendix 2: Quality Assurance Materials

QUALITY ASSURANCE

Day ____________________

Group Leader Plan

Quizzes

I. *Objectives*: Members will be able to:
   A. Prequiz: Demonstrate how much they currently know about each topic area.
   B. Postquiz: Demonstrate their ability to learn, store, and recall information particular to each topic.

II. *Materials*: Form A2-1, Form A2-2, Form A2-3, Form A2-4; Table A2-1, "Quality Assurance Data Sheet"; and group leader plans "Answers to Time Management Quiz," "Answers to Stress Management Quiz," "Answers to Social Skills Quiz," or "Answers to ADL Quiz."

III. *Procedures:*
   A. Quizzes are given twice for each topic area, once before the topic begins (prequiz) and the same quiz again after the topic is completed (postquiz). Form A2-1, "Time Management Quiz," Form A2-2, "Stress Management Quiz," Form A2-3, "Social Skills Quiz," Form A2-4, "Activities of Daily Living Quiz."
      1. Handout the quiz for the topic area you are beginning/completing.
      2. Allow time for completion.
   B. Grade quizzes by using the appropriate answer sheet.
      1. Divide total number correct by total number of questions and multiply by 100 to get the percentage correct.
      2. Record this percentage in the pretest or posttest column of Table A2-1, "Quality Assurance Data Sheet."

TIME MANAGEMENT

Day __________________

Group Leader Plan

Answers to Time Management Quiz

1. What is meant by "procrastination"?
   Putting off things that you need to do until later.
2. Name three techniques a person could use to better manage their time.
   a. Make lists of things that need to be done.
   b. Keep a calendar.
   c. Delegate work (ask for help).
   d. Prioritize what needs to be done.
   e. Plan ahead of time for the weekends.
   f. Know what your high, low, and medium levels of energy are.
   g. Wake up at the same time each morning and go to bed at the same time each night, eat three meals a day near the same time each day.
3. Why is it important to have a schedule?
   a. To plan ahead.
   b. To make more choices.
   c. To structure yourself.
   d. So you can complete all the things you need to get done.
   e. To avoid procrastination, which can lead to feeling overwhelmed.
   f. To know when you have time to do something with someone else.
   g. To see if you have a daily balance of work, play, and leisure activities.
4. Define:
   a. High energy times—the times of day when you have the most physical energy.
   b. Low energy activities—tasks which require a small amount of effort.
5. State three ways you could help yourself to get to appointments on time.
   a. Ask for a wake up call.
   b. Lay out your clothes the night before.
   c. Plan ahead of time by keeping a calendar and checking it daily.
   d. Buy a watch or find a clock in your area.
   e. Set an alarm.
6. List two ways drugs/alcohol have affected your time management skills.

This is a personal question, but examples may be drawn from the following:

a. Irregular sleep patterns.
b. Low energy.
c. Spending most of the time in drug-seeking behavior.
d. Decreased interest in leisure pursuits.
e. Less time spent with family and/or friends.

Time Management Quiz

1. What is meant by "procrastination"?

2. Name three techniques a person could use to better manage their time.

   a.

   b.

   c.

3. Why is it important to have a schedule?

4. Define:

   a. High energy times

   b. Low energy activities

5. State three ways you could help yourself get to appointments on time.

   a.

   b.

   c.

6. List two ways that drugs/alcohol have affected your time management skills.

STRESS MANAGEMENT

Day ____________________

Group Leader Plan

Answers to Stress Management Quiz

1. Define "stress."
   A physiological and psychological response to events which can be challenging, frustrating or overwhelming in nature.
2. List five stress management techniques:
   Deep breathing, exercise, warm bath, assertiveness, yoga, stretching, walking, time management, anger management, problem solving, goal setting, meditations, proper nutrition, playing or listening to music, biofeedback, hobbies/crafts.
3. List the five steps of goal setting:
   a. Identifying a problem.
   b. Writing a goal reflecting the problem.
   c. Stating why the goal is important.
   d. Listing four ways to achieve the goal.
   e. Executing the steps.
4. When can stress be helpful?
   In low amounts it can be motivating.
5. How do you react under stress?
   This is a personal question, but answers may be drawn from the following: sweaty palms, perspiration, heart palpitations, "butterflies" in stomach, muscle tension, headaches, shortness of breath, sore throat, fatigue, poor concentration, thought blocking, feeling overwhelmed, getting angry.
6. List two ways drugs/alcohol have affected your stress management skills. This is a personal question, but answers may be drawn from the following:
   a. Relied on drugs/alcohol to manage stress or deal with feelings.
   b. Once clean it's harder to deal with stress.
   c. Do not develop natural ways to deal with stress.
   d. Using drugs/alcohol creates more stress.

Stress Management Quiz*

1. Define "stress."

2. List five stress management techniques:
   a.
   b.
   c.
   d.
   e.

3. List the five steps of goal setting:
   a.
   b.
   c.
   d.
   e.

4. When can stress be helpful?

5. How do you react under stress? (List three reactions.)
   a.
   b.
   c.

6. List two ways drugs/alcohol have affected your stress management skills.
   a.
   b.

*Modified with permission from Schwimmer-Stern, P. Living Skills Curriculum (unpublished master's project), 1986.

SOCIAL SKILLS

Day ________________

Group Leader Plan

Answers to Social Skills Quiz

1. Define:
   a. Passive—not expressing your needs.
   b. Assertive—letting your needs be known without hurting anyone else physically or emotionally.
   c. Aggressive—expressing your needs in a way which *does* hurt someone either physically or emotionally.
2. List two techniques used to keep a conversation going:
   a. Talking about a topic you are familiar with.
   b. Open-ended questions.
   c. Body cues/body language (nods, “uhughs,” “yes”).
   d. Paraphrasing.
   e. Asking for clarification.
   f. Active listening.
3. What is a closed-ended question?
   A question which can be answered in one word.
4. List three ways to better adjust to change:
   a. Identify an upcoming change.
   b. Think of the worst thing that could happen.
   c. Picture yourself going through the change.
   d. Break the change into specific parts and deal with one at a time.
   e. Get help from someone else who has already gone through it.
   f. Communicate with someone who is going through it now.
   g. Give it up to your higher power.
   h. Take one step at a time.
5. What are the five steps of goal setting?
   a. Identifying a problem.
   b. Writing a goal reflecting the problem.
   c. State why the goal is important.
   d. List four steps to achieve the goal.
   e. Execute the steps.
6. List two ways that drugs/alcohol have affected your social skills. This is a personal question but examples may be drawn from the following:
   a. Lost friends.
   b. Lost family members.
   c. Kicked out of the house.
   d. Divorced/separated.

e. Lost custody of child.
f. Homeless or kicked out of a residence.
g. Arrested.
h. Stole from family/friends or others.
i. No clean friends.
j. Lonely, isolated.
k. Increasing arguments.
l. Physical fights.
m. Using.

Form A2-3

Social Skills Quiz

1. Define:

   a. Passive

   b. Assertive

   c. Aggressive

2. List two techniques used to keep a conversation going:

   a.

   b.

3. What is a closed-ended question?

4. List three ways to better adjust to change:

   a.

   b.

   c.

5. What are the five steps of goal setting?

   a.

   b.

   c.

   d.

   e.

6. List two ways that drugs/alcohol have affected your social skills:

   a.

   b.

ACTIVITIES OF DAILY LIVING

Day__________________

Group Leader Plan

Answers to Activities of Daily Living Quiz

1. List four examples of activities of daily living:
   a. Transportation.
   b. Hygiene.
   c. Money management.
   d. Home/Apartment maintenance.
   e. Nutrition.
   f. Work.
   g. Leisure.
2. List two bad effects that alcohol and drugs have on nutrition:
   a. Lack of vitamin B.
   b. Dehydration.
3. List two money management techniques:
   a. List expenditures.
   b. Total income.
   c. Budget money.
   d. Get a checking account.
   e. Ask for someone to keep your money for you.
   f. Get a savings account.
4. List three ways to improve hygiene:
   a. Brush teeth after each meal.
   b. Do laundry at least one time per week.
   c. Shower and shave daily.
5. List three skills that are necessary to maintain your own apartment/home:
   a. Cleaning.
   b. Budgeting.
   c. Washing dishes.
6. What are five steps of goal setting?
   a. Identifying a problem.
   b. Writing a goal reflecting the problem.
   c. Stating why the goal is important.
   d. Listing four ways to achieve the goal.
   e. Executing the steps.
7. List two ways that drugs/alcohol have affected your activities of daily living.
   This is a personal question but examples may be drawn from the following:
   a. Spent most of my money on drugs/alcohol.

b. Stopped eating on a regular basis.
c. Stopped bathing and washing my clothes.
d. Became homeless.
e. Could not manage my apartment.
f. Prostituted myself for drug money.
g. Spent most of my time in drug/alcohol-seeking behaviors.

Activities of Daily Living Quiz

1. List four examples of activities of daily living:
   a.
   b.
   c.
   d.
2. List two bad effects that alcohol and drugs have on nutrition:
   a.
   b.
3. List two money management techniques:
   a.
   b.
4. List three ways to improve hygiene:
   a.
   b.
   c.
5. List three skills that are necessary to maintain your own apartment/home:
   a.
   b.
   c.
6. What are the five steps in goal setting?
   a.
   b.
   c.
   d.
   e.
7. List two ways that drugs/alcohol have affected your activities of daily living:
   a.
   b.

ACTIVITIES OF DAILY LIVING

Day____________________

Group Leader Plan

Topic Evaluations

I. *Objectives*: Members will be able to:
   A. Give constructive feedback about each topic.

II. *Materials*: Form A2-5.

III. *Procedures*:
   A. Form A2-5, "Topic Evaluation."
      1. Have members complete the evaluation honestly, stating that their feedback will help you design further sessions to better meet their needs.
      2. Collect and record their results in the member report column (learned new material, made changes in life) of Table A2-1, "Quality Assurance Data Sheet."
      3. Tally up all members' responses to all questions and provide staff with results in percentages.

Topic Evaluation

1. I think this topic was ______________________.

   Very helpful   Somewhat helpful   Not helpful

2. I learned ______________________ from this topic.

   A lot   Some things   Nothing

3. I ______________________ recommend this topic to other members.

   Would   Would not

4. The thing I disliked about this topic was ______________________

   ______________________.

5. The think I liked most about this topic was ______________________

   ______________________.

6. I thought the group leader was ______________________.

   Clear   Not clear

7. This topic ______________________ help me make changes in my life outside the program.

   Did   Did not

ALL TOPICS

Day____________________

Group Leader Plan

Quality Assurance Data Sheet

1. *Objectives*: Group leader will be able to:
   A. Record each member's progress on a data sheet in numerical form.
   B. Ask and record staff's observations of client's progress during the time this group was in session.
   C. Determine whether or not the treatment was therapeutically effective and why or why not.
   D. Make necessary adjustments in future treatment to fit members' needs and levels of learning.

II. *Materials*: Table A2-1 and a calculator.

III. *Procedures*:
   A. Table A2-1, "Quality Assurance Data Sheet."
      1. Group leader completes as follows:
         a. Client—list member's initials or record number.
         b. Pretest—record the percentage of correct answers.
         c. Posttest—record the percentage of correct answers. The difference between the posttest and the pretest is a measure of how much new academic material the client was able to learn, memorize, and recall.
         d. Attendance—record the percentage of total days attended.
         e. Objectives met—go through each group leader plan and count the number of objectives that a particular member achieved throughout the duration of the group. This is best done if completed after each session for each member. The total score is then recorded in the form of the percentage of total objectives met (this measures the member's ability to understand and utilize the material presented in each group during the group).
         f. Goals met—record the number of goals each member achieved throughout the duration of the topic. This is a measure of how well the member was able to generalize newly learned material to his outside environment and use it appropriately with adequate problem solving skills.
         g. Member report:
            1. Learned new material—check here if members responded "yes" to question 2 in their Form A2-5, "Group Evaluation."

2. Made changes in life—check here if member reported "yes" to question 7 in their Form A2-5, "Group Evaluation."

h. Staff observations—ask other staff members what changes they have observed in the members. For example, in "Time Management," examples would be better use of break time, more punctual to program, able to tolerate full day of therapeutic activities, beginning to volunteer work, rehabilitation ready.

Table A2-1 Quality Assurance Data Sheet

Topic

						Member Report			
Client	*Pretest*	*Posttest*	*Attendance*	*Objectives Met*	*Goals Met*	*Learned New Material*	*Made Changes In Life*	*Staff Observations*	*Clean Time*

Glossary

Abstinence: To stay off drugs. "Complete abstinence" means to stay 100 percent drug free without a slip, a relapse, a binge, or without picking up at all.

Addiction: Someone is addicted to something when they can no longer control the amount of time spent doing it, and when it interferes with the most basic aspects of life. Addiction to a chemical substance (for example, drug) means that a person can no longer control their use of the drug even when it causes problems in their life. There may be psychological and/or physiological dependence on the substance.

Binge: To use large amounts of drugs over a short period of time. A binge may be preceded and followed by periods of clean time. If a binge is repeated over and over, it is called "bingeing."

Chemical abuse: The same as "substance abuse."

Clean: Refers to being drug free.

Clean friends: Friends who are not using drugs.

Clean time: The number of consecutive drug free days that a person has accumulated. If a person relapses, their clean time starts all over again.

Consumer: Someone who utilizes a service. For example, an MICA Consumer is someone who uses treatment for both substance abuse and mental illness.

Cravings: Urges to use drugs. They may or may not be acted on.

Denial: When someone does not fully see the extent to which they or someone they know is using drugs. When someone does not fully see the effects that drugs have on their life. The person in denial may underreport drug use and its effect on them. They may make excuses to themselves and others.

Double trouble: A treatment group which focuses on both substance abuse and mental illness.

Drug: A mood altering substance which may be addictive and/or illegal. The word *drug* when used in this book includes alcohol but does not include psychoactive prescription drugs used for the treatment of psychiatric illnesses.

Drug free hobbies: Enjoyable pursuits that do not involve any drug-related activities.

Drug money: Money used for buying drugs or money made in selling drugs.

Dual diagnosis: Having two diagnoses. In this book, *dual diagnosis* refers to having both a psychiatric illness and a substance abuse problem.

Harm reduction: The idea that complete abstinence may be unattainable, and a decrease in use is better than no clean time at all.

MICA (Mentally Ill Chemical Abuser): A chemical abuser is someone who abuses substances such as alcohol, crack, cocaine, heroin, amphetamines, or over-the-counter medication and meets the DSM IV criteria for substance abuse or dependence. Someone who is mentally ill meets any of the criteria for mental illness in the DSM IV Manual. A MICA consumer is a person who suffers from both a mental illness and substance abuse.

People, places, and things: A phrase referring to people who are using drugs, places where drugs are being used, and things that have to do drugs. A more common phrase that people use in recovery is "stay away from people, places, and things." It is believed that avoiding these three things will increase chances of sobriety.

Pick up: Refers to using drugs. For example, "Did you pick up today?"

Recovery: The lifelong process of becoming and remaining drug free.

Relapse: When a person uses drugs again after being clean.

Relapse prevention: The active work that is performed daily to remain drug free. It includes constant awareness of emotions, triggers, risky behaviors, and cravings. It also includes managing daily stress as it arises; dealing with anger; staying away from people, places, and things; and structuring time. It includes some form of help with the above, such as attending 12-step meetings, a dual diagnosis program, and/or community involvement.

Risky behavior: Behavior(s) which may lead to a relapse. People in recovery are usually advised to avoid risky behaviors. Examples may include walking through a neighborhood that is known for high drug traffic, missing 12-step meetings, or spending time with a partner who is actively using.

Slip: When someone with clean time uses again then stops using right away, the person is said to have had a "slip." Clean time begins from zero after a slip. People are encouraged to discuss their slips with their sponsor or counselor in order to admit having used again and to learn more about their pattern of addiction.

Sobriety: A state of clear thinking that results from being drug free.

Staying clean: Refers to staying off of drugs.

Substance abuse: The abuse or dependence on mood altering chemicals taken into the body such as alcohol, inhalants, crack, heroin, cocaine, barbiturates, amphetamines, and/or hallucinogens. Also called "chemical abuse."

Tokens: Rewards for clean time usually given after 30, 60, and 90 days, one year, and so on.

Triggers: Things that influence substance abusers to use a drug at that particular moment. For example, triggers can be thoughts (I do not deserve to be happy), feelings (anger), events (holidays), places (bars), people (old friends who still use drugs), situations (being fired from a job), things (money), or a combination of the above.

12-step: Guidelines to help people overcome addictive behaviors. There are 12 guidelines that progress in a stepwise fashion. Each step is to be "worked" before proceeding to the next.

Use: Refers to drug use.

Using: Refers to using drugs.

Index